The Art of Equilibrium

The Art of Equilibrium

Enhancing Balance and Coordination

Rafeal Mechlore

UNIEK ENTERPRISES

CONTENTS

INDEX

Chapter 1: The Importance of Balance and Coordination
1.1Introduction to the significance of balance and coordination.
1.2How they impact daily life and overall well-being.

Chapter 2: The Science Behind Balance
2.1Explanation of the physiological systems involved in balance.
2.2Factors affecting balance and potential risks.

Chapter 3: The Coordination Connection
3.1Defining coordination and its relationship to balance.
3.2The neurological basis of coordination.

Chapter 4: Assessing Your Current State
4.1Self-assessment tools and tests for balance and coordination.
4.2Identifying areas that need improvement.

Chapter 5: Enhancing Balance
5.1Physical exercises and training techniques for better balance.
5.2Lifestyle adjustments and nutritional considerations.

Chapter 6: Improving Coordination
6.1Coordination-building exercises and drills.
6.2Integrating coordination into daily activities.

Chapter 7: Lifespan Considerations
7.1Addressing balance and coordination in different life stages.
7.2Strategies for seniors to prevent falls and injuries.

Chapter 8: Achieving Balance in Life

8.1 Balancing work and personal life for overall equilibrium.
8.2 Stress management techniques for improved balance.

In the terrific woven artwork of life, equilibrium and coordination act as the imperceptible strings that wind around together our encounters, yearnings, and achievements. From the second we make our most memorable unstable strides as newborn children to the effortless developments of a talented artist, from the accuracy of a specialist's hand to the exquisite progression of a stunning musician, the specialty of harmony is a fundamental component in each feature of human life.

Envision a tightrope walker ready high over a clamoring cityscape, each stage a fragile dance among life and gravity. They exemplify the quintessence of equilibrium and coordination in its most instinctive structure. However, the harmony they show isn't restricted to the carnival tent or the stunt-devil's stage. It resounds all through our lives, forming our actual capacities, close to home prosperity, and, surprisingly, our progress in the complex fields of work, connections, and self-satisfaction.

In "The Specialty of Harmony: Improving Equilibrium and Coordination," we leave on an excursion into the domains of equilibrium and coordination, investigating the significant effect they use over the human experience. This book is a demonstration of the complex exchange of brain and body, offering experiences, methods, and shrewdness to assist you with dominating this creativity in your own life.

The Meaning of Equilibrium and Coordination

Equilibrium and coordination are not simple actual qualities; they are the cornerstones of usefulness and elegance. Without balance, we stagger through life, figuratively and straightforwardly. Our actual equilibrium keeps us upstanding, lessening the gamble of falls and wounds, and permits us to move easily through our current circumstance. In any case, balance stretches out past the actual domain. It likewise appears in the balance of our feelings, our connections, and our general prosperity.

Coordination, then again, is the amicable synchronization of our body's different parts. It empowers us to perform complex errands with artfulness, whether it's stringing a needle, spilling a b-ball, or composing a message on a console. Coordination is the director organizing the orchestra of our developments.

From the competitor taking a stab at maximized execution to the senior resident trying to keep up with freedom, from the craftsman consummating their art to the workplace laborer hoping to lessen the cost of a stationary way of life, the mission for further

developed equilibrium and coordination rises above age, occupation, and foundation. Fundamentally, it is an all inclusive quest for a higher condition.

The Motivation behind This Book

"The Craft of Harmony" is an exhaustive aide that dives profound into the workmanship and study of equilibrium and coordination. Our point is to demystify these complicated ideas, giving you a guide to upgrade your physical and mental harmony. Whether you are a competitor endeavoring to arrive at new levels, an understudy looking to further develop concentration and efficiency, or essentially somebody who wants to carry on with a more adjusted and amicable life, this book offers important bits of knowledge, down to earth works out, and a comprehensive way to deal with accomplishing your objectives.

Through the pages of this book, you will find the internal operations of your body's equilibrium frameworks, gain a more profound comprehension of the brain body association, and learn commonsense techniques to work on your equilibrium and coordination. In addition, you will come to see the value in the significant effect of balance on your general prosperity, and how it stretches out a long ways past the actual domain into the texture of your regular presence.

Our process together will incorporate the physiological, mental, and useful parts of equilibrium and coordination. It will furnish you with the devices to evaluate your present status, put forth sensible objectives, and carry out successful techniques for improving your harmony. In addition, it will investigate the job of equilibrium in different life stages, from adolescence to advanced age, and what it means for your capacity to succeed in the assorted fields of your life.

As we leave on this investigation of the craft of balance, we welcome you to open your brain and embrace the potential for change that exists in these pages. Toward the finish of this excursion, you won't just have a more profound comprehension of equilibrium and coordination yet additionally the commonsense abilities to dominate this masterfulness and apply it to each feature of your life. Welcome to "The Craft of Harmony."

Chapter 1

The Importance of Balance And Coordination

Equilibrium and coordination are major parts of human development and usefulness. They assume a significant part in our day to day routines, influencing our actual wellbeing, by and large prosperity, and, surprisingly, our progress in different exercises. In this investigation of the significance of equilibrium and coordination, we will dive profound into the physiological, mental, and viable parts of these fundamental abilities, understanding what they mean for us from youth to advanced age.

The Underpinnings of Equilibrium and Coordination

Equilibrium and coordination are two interrelated abilities that structure the underpinning of our actual capacities. In this section, we'll investigate the fundamentals of equilibrium and coordination and how they add to our general wellbeing and usefulness.

Figuring out Equilibrium

Balance is the capacity to keep up with harmony and stay stable in an upstanding position or while moving. It includes a perplexing interaction of tactile information, muscle strength, and engine control. We'll dive into the critical parts of equilibrium:

Tactile Info: The job of the vestibular framework, proprioception, and vision in keeping up with balance.

Muscle Strength: What muscle tone and strength mean for our capacity to remain upstanding.

Engine Control: The mind's job in handling tactile data and conveying messages to change our stance and development.

Unloading Coordination

Coordination is the consistent combination of various body parts to play out a particular undertaking. It incorporates many developments, from fine coordinated abilities like penmanship to net coordinated abilities like playing sports. We'll investigate:

Fine Engine Coordination: Abilities including little muscle gatherings, for example, dexterity for exact errands.

Gross Engine Coordination: Bigger developments like running, bouncing, and tossing that require composed exertion from different muscle gatherings.

The Mind's Job: How the cerebrum organizes developments by conveying messages to muscles in a planned way.

The Actual Advantages of Equilibrium and Coordination

Keeping up with actual wellbeing is perhaps of the clearest justification for why equilibrium and coordination are fundamental. These abilities are not restricted to forestalling falls yet in addition influence different parts of our actual prosperity.

Fall Counteraction

Falls can bring about serious wounds, particularly among the older. We'll examine how further developing equilibrium and coordination can fundamentally lessen the gamble of falls and breaks.

Injury Avoidance

Past falls, coordination assumes a significant part in physical issue counteraction across all age gatherings, especially in competitors and genuinely dynamic people. We'll investigate how better coordination can forestall sports-related wounds and different incidents.

Stance and Arrangement

Great stance is subject to adjust and coordination. We'll talk about how these abilities add to keeping up with appropriate stance, decreasing the gamble of outer muscle issues, and mitigating persistent agony.

Strength and Muscle Improvement

Solid, facilitated muscles are essential for day to day exercises and sports execution. We'll analyze how further developing coordination improves muscle advancement and strength.

The Mental Advantages of Equilibrium and Coordination

While frequently connected with actual ability, equilibrium and coordination likewise significantly affect mental capability and emotional well-being.

Cerebrum Wellbeing and Mental Capability

Adjusted developments and coordination animate cerebrum movement, adding to worked on mental capability, memory, and critical thinking abilities.

Stress Decrease

Actual work that includes equilibrium and coordination lessens pressure and uneasiness, advancing mental prosperity.

Concentration and Consideration

Better coordination upgrades the cerebrum's capacity to concentrate and support consideration, which is advantageous in different parts of life, including work and schooling.

Equilibrium and Coordination Across the Life expectancy

Equilibrium and coordination are abilities that advance as we age, making them significant contemplations in various life stages.

Youth Improvement

We'll investigate how equilibrium and coordination foster in kids and why these abilities are urgent for their physical and mental development.

Adulthood and Efficiency

In adulthood, equilibrium and coordination keep on being fundamental, influencing work execution, actual wellness, and by and large prosperity.

Seniors and Autonomy

As we age, keeping up with equilibrium and coordination becomes basic for keeping up with autonomy and forestalling falls.

Equilibrium and Coordination in Sports and Wellness

Competitors and wellness devotees depend vigorously on equilibrium and coordination for progress in their picked exercises.

Athletic Execution

We'll talk about how competitors from different games rely upon exact coordination and adjust to succeed in their disciplines.

Wellness and Exercise

Whether in the exercise center or during outside exercises, coordination assumes a significant part in upgrading exercises and staying away from wounds.

Down to earth Ways to further develop Equilibrium and Coordination

Understanding the significance of equilibrium and coordination is just the initial step. This section gives down to earth tips and activities to upgrading these abilities.

Equilibrium Activities

We'll investigate a scope of equilibrium practices that can be integrated into everyday schedules to further develop strength.

Coordination Drills

Different drills and exercises pointed toward upgrading coordination will be examined, offering perusers noteworthy stages to improve their abilities.

Incorporating Equilibrium and Coordination into Day to day existence

To genuinely see the value in the significance of equilibrium and coordination, we should figure out how to coordinate them flawlessly into our day to day schedules.

Way of life Changes

We'll talk about way of life changes that can advance better equilibrium and coordination, from dietary acclimations to rest and stress the executives.

The Brain Body Association

Investigating how mental practices like care and representation can improve actual equilibrium and coordination.

The Continuous Excursion of Equilibrium and Coordination

The significance of equilibrium and coordination isn't restricted to a specific phase of life or a solitary part of wellbeing; it's a long lasting excursion.

Putting forth and Arriving at Objectives

Grasping the significance of continuous improvement and the benefit of setting and accomplishing equilibrium and coordination objectives.

Past the Physical

Investigating the more extensive ramifications of equilibrium and coordination in private and expert achievement, as well as in accomplishing a healthy lifestyle.

1.1 Introduction to the significance of balance and coordination.

Equilibrium and coordination are two major mainstays of human actual ability. They are frequently underestimated until they become compromised, yet their importance resounds through each aspect of our lives, from our day to day schedules to our most aggressive undertakings. These abilities are so fundamental to our prosperity that we frequently neglect their significance until we experience hardships or provokes that compel us to deal with their nonappearance. In this investigation of the meaning of equilibrium and coordination, we will dive profound into their complex jobs, understanding what they mean for our wellbeing, execution, and generally speaking personal satisfaction.

The Quintessence of Equilibrium

In our excursion through the meaning of equilibrium and coordination, we start with the establishment, balance. Balance is the capacity to keep a steady and upstanding position, whether fixed or moving.

This expertise is so profoundly imbued in our regular routines that we seldom require some investment to see the value in its intricacy and significance.

The Pervasiveness of Equilibrium

Balance isn't bound to the domain of tumblers and gymnasts; it is an expertise we depend on from the second we figure out how to remain on two feet. We'll investigate how equilibrium is a steady presence in our lives, from strolling and climbing steps to absolutely getting up.

The Physiology of Equilibrium

The capacity to adjust is a wonder of human science. We'll dive into the complex frameworks that add to our feeling of equilibrium, including:

The Vestibular Framework: Situated in the internal ear, this framework assumes a focal part in recognizing changes in head position and development.

Proprioception: The body's natural feeling of its own situation in space, which contributes essentially to adjust.

Visual Info: How our eyes give basic data to assist us with keeping up with balance.

Equilibrium and Fall Anticipation

One of the most prompt and substantial parts of equilibrium is its job in fall anticipation. Falls can have crushing results, particularly in more seasoned grown-ups. We'll talk about the connection among equilibrium and fall avoidance, and how further developing equilibrium can lessen the gamble of falls and related wounds.

The Intricacy of Coordination

As we push ahead in our investigation, we experience coordination — an expertise that supplements and frequently covers with balance. Coordination is the specialty of easily and effectively incorporating different body parts to perform explicit assignments. It incorporates many developments, from the exact and fragile to the strong and strong.

The Exchange of Muscles and Joints

Coordination depends on the amicable participation of muscles and joints. We'll dig into how the body organizes these developments through perplexing brain signs and criticism components.

Fine Engine Coordination

Fine coordinated abilities include the utilization of little muscle gatherings and exact developments. We'll investigate how these abilities are urgent in exercises like penmanship, playing instruments, and in any event, composing on a console.

Gross Engine Coordination

On the opposite finish of the range, gross coordinated abilities include huge muscle gatherings and greater developments. We'll examine how coordination assumes a crucial part in sports, dance, and other genuinely requesting exercises.

The Association Between Equilibrium, Coordination, and Generally Prosperity

Equilibrium and coordination are not disengaged abilities — they are interconnected with our generally physical and mental prosperity. In this part, we investigate the comprehensive idea of these abilities.

Actual Wellbeing

Our actual wellbeing is significantly impacted by equilibrium and coordination. We'll examine what these abilities mean for injury avoidance, act, muscle strength, and that's just the beginning.

Mental Capability

The connection between actual development and mental capability is an interesting one. We'll investigate how further developing equilibrium and coordination can improve mind wellbeing, memory, and critical thinking skills.

Stress Decrease and Profound Prosperity

Active work that includes equilibrium and coordination can affect the brain. We'll dive into how these exercises can assist with diminishing pressure, uneasiness, and work on close to home prosperity.

The Job of Equilibrium and Coordination Across the Life expectancy

Equilibrium and coordination are abilities that advance and adjust as we progress through various phases of life. From youth to advanced age, they assume exceptional parts in forming our turn of events and in general personal satisfaction.

Adolescence Improvement

In adolescence, equilibrium and coordination are fundamental for physical and mental turn of events. We'll investigate how these abilities impact the development of youngsters and why early improvement is vital.

Adulthood and Efficiency

In adulthood, equilibrium and coordination keep on assuming a urgent part in keeping up with actual wellness, work environment efficiency, and in general prosperity. We'll examine how these abilities add to progress in different parts of grown-up life.

Seniors and Freedom

As we age, keeping up with equilibrium and coordination turns out to be significantly more basic. Falls can have serious ramifications for seniors. We'll investigate procedures for seniors to safeguard their freedom and forestall falls.

Equilibrium and Coordination in Sports and Wellness

Competitors and wellness lovers are personally acquainted with the significance of equilibrium and coordination. In this section, we'll dig into how these abilities are central in the realm of sports and actual wellness.

Athletic Execution

Competitors from various games depend on exact coordination and equilibrium for progress. We'll investigate how these abilities become possibly the most important factor in different athletic disciplines.

Wellness and Exercise

Coordination isn't just for competitors but on the other hand is basic for those seeking after broad wellness and exercise. We'll talk about how further developing coordination can improve exercises and diminish the gamble of wounds.

Down to earth Ways to upgrade Equilibrium and Coordination

Understanding the meaning of equilibrium and coordination is just the start. This part offers viable guidance and activities to assist people with working on these abilities.

Equilibrium Activities

We'll investigate a scope of equilibrium practices that can be integrated into everyday schedules to improve steadiness and diminish the gamble of falls.

Coordination Drills

Different drills and exercises pointed toward upgrading coordination will be talked about, offering perusers noteworthy stages to work on their abilities.

Incorporating Equilibrium and Coordination into Day to day existence

Equilibrium and coordination are not abilities held for explicit exercises or minutes; they ought to be consistently incorporated into our regular routines.

Way of life Changes

We'll examine way of life changes that can advance better equilibrium and coordination, including dietary changes, rest examples, and stress the executives procedures.

The Brain Body Association

The association between mental practices like care and perception and worked on actual equilibrium and coordination will be investigated.

The Continuous Excursion of Equilibrium and Coordination

At last, we finish up our investigation by underscoring that the meaning of equilibrium and coordination isn't bound to a specific life stage or restricted to a particular part of wellbeing; it's a deep rooted venture.

Defining and Arriving at Objectives

Perceiving the significance of persistent improvement and the benefit of setting and accomplishing equilibrium and coordination objectives.

The More extensive Ramifications

Understanding that equilibrium and coordination reach out a long ways past actual abilities, impacting our own and proficient achievement, and adding to a healthy lifestyle.

1.2How they impact daily life and overall well-being.

Equilibrium and coordination, two apparently basic abilities, affect our day to day routines and in general prosperity. These capacities are fundamental for keeping up with actual wellbeing, advancing mental clearness, and accomplishing a feeling of congruity in our schedules. While they might be underestimated while working ideally, their importance ends up being obvious when compromised. In this investigation, we will dig into the multifaceted manners by which equilibrium and coordination impact our everyday presence and add to our all encompassing prosperity.

Equilibrium and Coordination in Ordinary Exercises

To really get a handle on the significance of equilibrium and coordination, perceiving their ubiquity in our day to day activities is fundamental. From the second we ascend in the first part of the day to the time we resign around evening time, these abilities are at play in manners we could not necessarily deliberately recognize.

Wake-up routines

We'll begin our excursion with the earliest reference point of the day — getting up, standing, and strolling to the washroom. Indeed, even these apparently commonplace assignments include equilibrium and coordination.

Day to day Tasks

From planning breakfast to cleaning up, cooking, and cleaning, equilibrium and coordination are fundamental for moving proficiently and securely through family tasks.

Driving and Transportation

For the people who drive to work or travel day to day, balance is vital while exploring swarmed trains, transports, or in any event, driving a vehicle. Coordination is likewise fundamental for errands like working a vehicle.

The Actual Advantages of Equilibrium and Coordination

While we may not necessarily in all cases acknowledge it, equilibrium and coordination are basic for keeping up with our actual wellbeing. These abilities act as an establishment for forestalling wounds and enhancing our actual capacities.

Fall Avoidance

Falls can have serious results, especially for more established grown-ups. We'll investigate how further developed equilibrium can altogether diminish the gamble of falls, cracks, and related wounds.

Injury Avoidance in Sports and Actual work

In sports and actual work, coordination is essential for forestalling wounds. Competitors depend on exact developments to succeed in their picked disciplines, and an absence of coordination can prompt mishaps.

Stance and Arrangement

Equilibrium and coordination are unpredictably connected to act. We'll talk about how keeping up with legitimate stance is essential for decreasing the gamble of outer muscle issues and lightening constant torment.

Strength and Muscle Improvement

Solid, facilitated muscles are fundamental for day to day exercises and sports execution. We'll investigate how further developed coordination upgrades muscle advancement and by and large strength.

The Mental Advantages of Equilibrium and Coordination

Our actual capacities and intellectual capacities are profoundly interwoven. Equilibrium and coordination likewise apply a significant effect on our mental capability and mental prosperity.

Mind Wellbeing and Mental Capability

Actual work that includes equilibrium and coordination animates cerebrum movement. We'll dig into how this excitement upgrades mental capability, memory, and critical thinking abilities.

Stress Decrease and Close to home Prosperity

Equilibrium and coordination exercises affect the brain. We'll investigate how these exercises assist with decreasing pressure, uneasiness, and advance profound prosperity.

Concentration and Consideration

Upgraded coordination additionally means further developed concentration and consideration. This has suggestions for different parts of life, including work and schooling.

Equilibrium and Coordination Across the Life expectancy

The meaning of equilibrium and coordination develops as we progress through various life stages. From youth to advanced age, these abilities assume unmistakable parts in our turn of events and in general personal satisfaction.

Adolescence Advancement

We'll investigate how equilibrium and coordination are fundamental for the physical and mental advancement of youngsters. Early improvement in these abilities makes way for a sound future.

Adulthood and Efficiency

In adulthood, equilibrium and coordination keep on being crucial. They influence efficiency in the working environment, actual wellness, and by and large prosperity. We'll examine how these abilities add to progress in different parts of grown-up life.

Seniors and Autonomy

As we age, keeping up with equilibrium and coordination turns out to be considerably more basic. Falls can have serious ramifications for seniors. We'll investigate procedures for protecting freedom and forestalling falls.

Equilibrium and Coordination in Sports and Wellness

Competitors and wellness aficionados are keenly conscious about the significance of equilibrium and coordination. In this part, we'll dig into how these abilities are foremost in sports and actual wellness.

Athletic Execution

Competitors from various games depend on exact coordination and equilibrium for progress. We'll investigate how these abilities become possibly the most important factor in different athletic disciplines.

Wellness and Exercise

Coordination isn't just for competitors however is basic for those chasing after broad wellness and exercise. We'll talk about how further developing coordination can advance exercises and decrease the gamble of wounds.

Functional Ways to upgrade Equilibrium and Coordination

Understanding the meaning of equilibrium and coordination is just the start. This part offers pragmatic counsel and activities to assist people with working on these abilities.

Equilibrium Activities

We'll investigate a scope of equilibrium practices that can be integrated into day to day schedules to improve dependability and decrease the gamble of falls.

Coordination Drills

Different drills and exercises pointed toward upgrading coordination will be examined, offering perusers noteworthy stages to work on their abilities.

Incorporating Equilibrium and Coordination into Day to day existence

Equilibrium and coordination ought not be segregated abilities however consistently incorporated into our day to day schedules. In this section, we'll examine how to make these abilities a characteristic piece of day to day existence.

Way of life Changes

We'll investigate way of life changes that can advance better equilibrium and coordination, including dietary changes, rest examples, and stress the board procedures.

The Psyche Body Association

The association between mental practices like care and representation and worked on actual equilibrium and coordination will be analyzed.

The Continuous Excursion of Equilibrium and Coordination

At long last, we close our investigation by underscoring that the meaning of equilibrium and coordination is a deep rooted venture, not bound to a particular life stage or part of wellbeing.

Laying out and Arriving at Objectives

Perceiving the significance of persistent improvement and the benefit of setting and accomplishing equilibrium and coordination objectives.

The More extensive Ramifications

Understanding that equilibrium and coordination reach out a long ways past actual abilities, impacting individual and expert achievement, and adding to a healthy lifestyle.

Chapter 2

The Science Behind Balance

Balance is an apparently straightforward demonstration, underestimated until we waver on the edge of a fall or endeavor a difficult actual accomplishment. However, underneath this obvious straightforwardness lies a multifaceted trap of tangible frameworks, brain processes, and outer muscle collaborations that permit us to stand upstanding, move with accuracy, and explore our general surroundings. The science behind balance is a captivating excursion into the inward operations of the human body and psyche. It envelops the vestibular framework, proprioception, visual info, and the mind's job in handling this tangible data. In this investigation, we'll leave on a journey through these striking systems, uncovering the secrets that empower us to keep up with balance and how this information can work on our lives.

The Underpinnings of Equilibrium

Balance, in its embodiment, is the capacity to keep a steady and upstanding position, whether fixed or moving. This expertise, essential to our regular routines, is unpredictably connected to the physiological frameworks that administer our bodies. At its center, balance includes a fragile exchange between tangible info, muscle strength, and engine control. Understanding these fundamental perspectives is fundamental to fathoming the science behind balance.

Characterizing Equilibrium

To investigate the study of equilibrium, we should initially characterize what equilibrium implies. It's the shortfall of falling as well as the dynamic course of keeping up with steadiness and balance. This act includes recognizing shifts ready and making ongoing acclimations to neutralize them, frequently happening without cognizant idea.

The Omnipresence of Equilibrium

Balance is universal in our regular routines. From standing up in the first part of the day to strolling, running, or just going after an article, we depend on balance ceaselessly. It is an uncelebrated yet truly great individual, supporting us in even the most everyday assignments.

The Vestibular Framework: Our Internal Equilibrium Compass

The vestibular framework, arranged inside our internal ear, is frequently alluded to as our "inward equilibrium compass." This complex tangible framework assumes a focal part in identifying changes in head position and development, contributing fundamentally to our feeling of equilibrium.

The Life structures of the Vestibular Framework

At the core of the vestibular framework are the crescent trenches and otolith organs, each with a particular job in identifying head developments. These designs, however little, are wonders of designing, permitting us to see changes in direction and change our stance in like manner.

Vestibular Capability in real life

Understanding how the vestibular framework capabilities is essential in getting a handle on the study of equilibrium. It distinguishes head developments, interprets their course and speed, and sends this data to the mind for handling. This quick hand-off of data empowers us to keep up with balance in any event, during fast or startling changes moving.

Vestibular Problems and Their Effect

Like any framework in the body, the vestibular framework can be helpless to problems and brokenness. These issues can appear in different ways, from dizziness and dazedness to disabled balance and spatial direction. Investigating these difficulties highlights the significance of a sound vestibular framework for ordinary harmony.

Proprioception: The Body's Inner GPS

Proprioception, frequently alluded to as our "intuition," is a fundamental supporter of our feeling of equilibrium. This inner GPS framework gives ongoing criticism about the position and development of our body parts, empowering us to make exact changes in accordance with keep up with harmony.

What Is Proprioception?

Proprioception is the tangible familiarity with our body's situation and development. It depends on particular receptors called proprioceptors, which are dissipated all through muscles, ligaments, and joints. These receptors constantly convey messages to the mind about the body's state in space.

Proprioception in Muscles and Joints

To fathom the study of equilibrium, we should dig into how proprioception capabilities inside muscles and joints. Proprioceptors in these tissues recognize factors like muscle length, pressure, and joint point. This data educates the cerebrum regarding appendage positions, taking into account exact changes.

Proprioception and Equilibrium

Proprioception and equilibrium are indistinguishable. Proprioceptors give the mind the data expected to make quick changes in muscle tone and joint development, keeping up with balance during exercises like strolling, running, or in any event, stopping.

Visual Info: Our Eyes as Equilibrium Helps

Our feeling of vision is one more critical supporter of equilibrium. Visual info gives fundamental data that assists us with keeping up with harmony by identifying changes in our environmental elements and giving spatial signs.

The Job of Vision in Equilibrium

Visual information assumes a critical part in balance. It gives us data about the climate, like the slant of the ground, the presence of obstructions, and the direction of articles. Our mind coordinates this visual information with input from other tactile frameworks to change act and keep up with strength.

Visual Info and Compensatory Methodologies

At the point when equilibrium is tested, our mind depends on visual contribution to make fast compensatory changes. This includes recognizing errors between what we see and what we feel, empowering us to address our stance and forestall falls.

Visual Unsettling influences and Equilibrium Issues

Disturbances to visual information, like visual disabilities or changes in the visual field, can significantly affect balance. Understanding what these aggravations mean for balance features the unpredictable job of vision in our capacity to remain upstanding.

The Cerebrum's Job in Handling Equilibrium Data

The mind fills in as the war room for handling tangible information connected with balance. This brain handling includes complex components, including sensorimotor coordination, engine control, and the urgent job of the cerebellum in calibrating our feeling of balance.

Sensorimotor Combination

The mind flawlessly coordinates tangible data from the vestibular framework, proprioception, and vision. This mix makes a thorough image of our body's situation in space, empowering us to make split-second changes.

Engine Control and Equilibrium

The cerebrum's engine control focuses get this coordinated tangible info and convey messages to muscles all through the body. These signs direct changes in muscle tone, stance, and appendage developments, permitting us to keep up with balance.

The Cerebellum: The Mind's Equilibrium Maestro

The cerebellum, a surprising design situated at the foundation of the cerebrum, assumes an imperative part in calibrating equilibrium and coordination. This little yet complex locale goes about as a maestro, coordinating exact developments and acclimations to keep us stable.

Normal Elements Influencing Equilibrium

Balance is certainly not a static expertise; it very well may be impacted by different variables, both inner and outer. This part investigates the normal factors that influence equilibrium and what they can mean for our regular routines.

Maturing and Equilibrium

As we age, keeping up with equilibrium can turn out to be seriously difficult. Changes in tactile discernment, muscle strength, and mental capability can influence harmony. We'll investigate the science behind these age-related changes and systems to moderate them.

Ailments and Equilibrium

Certain ailments, for example, inward ear problems or neurological circumstances, can disturb equilibrium and coordination. Understanding what these circumstances mean for the basic study of equilibrium is vital for compelling administration and treatment.

Meds and Equilibrium

A few drugs can have secondary effects that influence equilibrium and coordination. Diving into the science behind these impacts assists people with arriving at informed conclusions about their drugs and screen their equilibrium.

The Down to earth Utilization of Equilibrium Science

Understanding the science behind balance isn't simply a scholastic pursuit — it has useful ramifications for our regular routines. In this section, we overcome any issues among hypothesis and work on, examining how this information can be applied to upgrade equilibrium and generally prosperity.

Equilibrium Activities and Preparing

Investigating a scope of activities and preparing procedures pointed toward further developing equilibrium and coordination. These reasonable uses of equilibrium science engage people to improve their soundness and lessen the gamble of falls.

Fall Counteraction Systems

Examining systems and changes that can assist with diminishing the gamble of falls, especially in more established grown-ups. These systems are established in a comprehension of the study of equilibrium and its job in fall avoidance.

Equilibrium Appraisal Apparatuses

Investigating devices and tests that medical services experts use to survey a singular's equilibrium. These appraisals are grounded in the standards of equilibrium science and assist with distinguishing regions for development.

2.1 Explanation of the physiological systems involved in balance.

Balance, the capacity to keep an upstanding and stable position, is a mind boggling expertise that depends on an ensemble of physiological frameworks working as one. This mind boggling exchange includes the vestibular framework, proprioception, visual info, and the cerebrum's focal job in handling tactile data. Understanding the physiological systems behind balance is significant for forestalling falls and wounds as well as for streamlining execution in different proactive tasks. In this far reaching investigation, we will take apart every one of these physiological frameworks, divulging the momentous science that underlies our capacity to remain predictable on our feet.

The Vestibular Framework

The vestibular framework, arranged inside the inward ear, fills in as our body's interior equilibrium compass. This perplexing tangible framework assumes a focal part in distinguishing changes in head position and development, contributing fundamentally to our feeling of equilibrium.

The Life structures of the Vestibular Framework

The vestibular framework includes the half circle channels and otolith organs, each with an unmistakable design and capability.

Understanding the life structures of these parts is vital for handle their job in balance.

Vestibular Capability in real life

This segment dives into how the vestibular framework recognizes head developments and passes this data on to the cerebrum. It features the continuous changes it works with to keep up with balance during different exercises.

Vestibular Problems and Their Effect

Investigating normal vestibular problems, their side effects, and what they mean for balance highlights the meaning of a sound vestibular framework for harmony and day to day existence.

Proprioception: The Body's Inside GPS

Proprioception, frequently alluded to as our "intuition," gives constant criticism about the position and development of our body parts. This interior GPS framework empowers us to make exact acclimations to keep up with balance.

What Is Proprioception?

Characterizing proprioception and recognizing it from different faculties, like touch and vision, lays the basis for grasping its job in balance.

Proprioception in Muscles and Joints

Investigating how proprioceptors in muscles, ligaments, and joints capability. These receptors identify factors like muscle length, strain, and joint point, furnishing the cerebrum with basic data about appendage position.

Proprioception and Equilibrium

This part dives into how proprioception is indivisible from balance. Proprioceptors persistently convey messages to the cerebrum, empowering fast changes in muscle tone, joint development, and stance to keep up with balance.

Visual Info: Our Eyes as Equilibrium Helps

Vision assumes a vital part in balance by giving fundamental data about our environmental factors and spatial signals. This part investigates how visual information upholds our feeling of harmony.

The Job of Vision in Equilibrium

Analyzing the connection between visual information and equilibrium, remembering how it helps for recognizing changes in the climate, like slant, deterrents, and article direction.

Visual Info and Compensatory Methodologies

How the cerebrum utilizes visual contribution to make quick compensatory changes when equilibrium is tested, including distinguishing inconsistencies among visual and proprioceptive signs.

Visual Aggravations and Equilibrium Issues

Understanding what visual impedances or aggravations can significantly mean for balance, featuring the multifaceted job of vision in our capacity to keep up with solidness.

The Cerebrum's Part in Handling Equilibrium Data

The cerebrum fills in as the headquarters place for handling tactile info connected with balance. This part investigates the brain components included, including sensorimotor incorporation, engine control, and the meaning of the cerebellum.

Sensorimotor Incorporation

Investigating how the cerebrum coordinates tactile data from the vestibular framework, proprioception, and vision to make an exhaustive image of our body's situation in space. This incorporation is basic for making exact changes.

Engine Control and Equilibrium

Understanding how the cerebrum conveys messages to muscles all through the body, directing changes in muscle tone, stance, and appendage developments. This segment features the cerebrum's part in keeping up with balance.

The Cerebellum: The Cerebrum's Equilibrium Maestro

Diving into the vital job of the cerebellum in adjusting equilibrium and coordination. This little yet complex mind locale goes about as a maestro, coordinating exact developments and acclimations to keep us stable.

2.2 Factors affecting balance and potential risks.

Balance, the capacity to keep an upstanding and stable position, is a principal part of human capability that frequently slips through the cracks until it's compromised. Many elements can impact a singular's equilibrium, either briefly or persistently

Understanding these variables and their potential dangers is urgent for forestalling falls, wounds, and keeping up with by and large prosperity. In this exhaustive investigation, we will dig into the complex universe of equilibrium, analyzing age-related changes, ailments, drugs, natural elements, way of life decisions, and mental variables that can affect one's capacity to remain consistent on their feet.

Age-Related Changes and Equilibrium

As people age, they go through physiological changes that can altogether influence their equilibrium and increment the gamble of falls.

Tangible Changes

Age-related changes in tactile frameworks, including reduced vestibular capability (internal ear equilibrium) and proprioception (familiarity with body position), can think twice about person's capacity to distinguish shifts ready and make quick acclimations to keep up with balance.

Muscle Strength and Mass

Sarcopenia, the age-related loss of bulk and strength, can prompt decreased dependability and an expanded gamble of falls. Debilitating muscles make it harder to control development and keep up with harmony.

Mental Capability

Mental deterioration, normal in maturing, can influence a singular's capacity to handle tactile info, pursue fast choices, and respond to changes in balance. This disability in mental capability can expand the gamble of falls, particularly in mind boggling or new conditions.

Postural Changes

Age-related changes in stance and walk, frequently saw in more established grown-ups, can adjust the body's focal point of gravity and weight conveyance. These progressions can make it more testing to keep up with balance, particularly during strolling and other powerful exercises.

Ailments and Their Effect on Equilibrium

Different medical issue can by implication affect a singular's equilibrium and posture expected dangers to their prosperity.

Inward Ear Problems

Conditions like Meniere's illness or harmless paroxysmal positional dizziness (BPPV) can upset the vestibular framework, prompting unsteadiness and weakened balance. These inward ear issues can influence people, everything being equal.

Neurological Issues

Neurological circumstances like Parkinson's sickness, numerous sclerosis, or fringe neuropathy can influence the focal sensory system or fringe nerves, prompting balance issues. These circumstances frequently require particular administration and recovery.

Muscular Circumstances

Muscular circumstances, including osteoarthritis, joint torment, and outer muscle issues, can block portability and steadiness, essentially influencing balance. Persistent joint agony or versatility impediments might require versatile guides and exercise based recuperation.

Cardiovascular Issues

Hypotension (low pulse), arrhythmias, or other cardiovascular issues can prompt swooning or tipsiness, expanding the gamble of falls. Cardiovascular wellbeing assumes a pivotal part in keeping up with balance, stressing the significance of customary clinical check-ups.

Prescriptions and Their Consequences for Equilibrium

Certain drugs have incidental effects that can affect a singular's equilibrium, making it fundamental for people and medical care suppliers to know about expected chances.

Meds Influencing the Vestibular Framework

A few prescriptions, for example, those utilized for sensitivities, movement disorder, or dizziness, can influence the inward ear or vestibular framework, prompting discombobulation or dizziness. Understanding these potential secondary effects is fundamental for overseeing medicine regimens.

Meds Influencing Mental Capability

Prescriptions that influence mental capability, including tranquilizers, antipsychotics, or allergy meds, can hinder independent direction and coordination. These impacts can upset a singular's capacity to keep up with balance, particularly when these prescriptions are utilized simultaneously.

Prescriptions Influencing Muscle Capability

Certain meds, for example, muscle relaxants or medications with muscle-debilitating incidental effects, can think twice about person's capacity to help their body weight and keep up with steadiness.

Natural Factors and Equilibrium Dangers

The actual climate wherein people live and work can essentially influence their equilibrium and posture likely dangers.

Lopsided Surfaces

Strolling on lopsided surfaces, like rock ways or cold walkways, builds the gamble of outings and falls. Open air conditions, specifically, can introduce difficulties for balance.

Unfortunate Lighting

Deficient lighting can darken snags and risks, making it trying to keep up with balance and stay away from mishaps, particularly in faintly lit indoor spaces.

Jumbled Spaces

Jumbled living spaces or workspaces can prompt excursions and falls, particularly for more established grown-ups with diminished readiness. Keeping up with clear, coordinated spaces is fundamental for lessening such dangers.

Dangerous Floors

Wet or dangerous floors, whether because of spills or deficient foothold, represent a critical gamble to adjust. Such conditions request mindful route to forestall falls.

Way of life Decisions and Equilibrium

Individual way of life decisions, including diet, active work, substance use, and rest designs, can influence equilibrium and in general prosperity.

Diet and Sustenance

Nourishing decisions can influence bone wellbeing, muscle strength, and generally essentialness, which are all basic for balance. Satisfactory admission of supplements like calcium and vitamin D is fundamental for keeping up with bone wellbeing.

Active work

Customary active work, including balance works out, can reinforce muscles, further develop coordination, and upgrade by and large security. Taking part in suitable proactive tasks can assist with relieving balance-related gambles.

Liquor and Substance Use

Unreasonable liquor utilization or medication use can hinder mental capability and engine coordination, prompting balance issues. Familiarity with the impacts of substances on balance is critical for injury counteraction.

Rest and Weakness

Insufficient rest and persistent weakness can upset mental capability and increment the gamble of falls. Focusing on sound rest designs is fundamental for keeping up with ideal equilibrium and generally prosperity.

Mental Factors and Equilibrium

Mental elements, like pressure, tension, and feeling of dread toward falling, can influence a singular's certainty and equilibrium.

Stress and Nervousness

Constant pressure and nervousness can prompt muscle strain and changed act, influencing balance. Stress the executives strategies and care practices can assist with decreasing these impacts.

Anxiety toward Falling

People who have encountered falls or wounds might foster a feeling of dread toward falling, prompting diminished actual work and, thusly, more fragile equilibrium. Tending to this trepidation through treatment or support can be fundamental for recapturing trust in one's equilibrium capacities.

Techniques for Keeping up with and Improving Equilibrium

This section talks about different systems and intercessions pointed toward alleviating the impacts of variables that adversely influence balance.

Falls Avoidance Projects

Falls counteraction programs survey a singular's gamble factors for falling and give custom-made mediations, activities, and training to lessen those dangers. These projects are particularly valuable for more established grown-ups.

Non-intrusive treatment and Recovery

Non-intrusive treatment and recovery programs are intended to further develop strength, coordination, and equilibrium, frequently through designated activities and exercises.

Assistive Gadgets and Changes

Assistive gadgets, like sticks, walkers, or get bars, can upgrade security and decrease balance-related gambles, especially for those with portability challenges. Home alterations, such as introducing handrails or non-slip surfaces, can establish more secure residing conditions.

Chapter 3

The Coordination Connection

Coordination is a peculiarity that saturates each part of our lives, from the apparently basic demonstration of making a move to the multifaceted developments of a professional piano player's fingers. It is the ensemble of our muscles, nerves, and cerebrum working as one to accomplish exact and deliberate activities. This coordination association isn't restricted to actual developments alone; it stretches out into mental capabilities, social cooperations, and, surprisingly, our close to home prosperity. In this exhaustive investigation, we will dive into the complex universe of coordination, taking apart its physiological and neurological underpinnings, its mental and profound aspects, and its importance in different parts of life.

The Wonder of Strong Coordination

Coordination starts at the most key level with the synchronization of muscles, permitting us to perform even the easiest assignments with effortlessness and accuracy.

Muscle Constriction and Coordination

The complexities of muscle compression, from the sliding fiber hypothesis to the job of engine units, are key to understanding how muscles cooperate as a unified whole.

Fine Coordinated abilities and Sensitive Equilibrium

Fine coordinated abilities, from stringing a needle to playing an instrument, feature the fragile equilibrium of solid coordination expected for undertakings that request accuracy and skill.

Gross Coordinated movements and Athletic Ability

Investigating gross coordinated abilities grandstands the job of coordination in athletic execution, from running to vaulting, and how competitors bridle their bodies' coordination for uncommon accomplishments.

The Neurological Wiring of Coordination

Behind each organized development is a perplexing trap of brain processes and signals coordinating the whole ensemble. Understanding the neurological premise of coordination is urgent.

The Focal Sensory system's Control

Digging into the job of the focal sensory system, especially the mind and spinal string, in planning developments and activities.

Tangible Criticism and Engine Control

Looking at how tactile criticism, like proprioception and vision, assumes a pivotal part in illuminating the cerebrum and changing developments to accomplish coordination.

Engine Learning and Muscle Memory

Revealing the systems of engine advancing and how our minds lay out muscle memory to perform complex activities with expanding productivity.

The Mental Components of Coordination

Coordination stretches out past the actual domain and into the mental space, where arranging, consideration, and direction are central participants.

Chief Capabilities and Arranging

Investigating the leader elements of the cerebrum, including arranging and association, and how they are fundamental for planning complex activities.

Consideration and Concentration

The job of consideration and concentration in organizing activities, from driving a vehicle in weighty rush hour gridlock to dominating a melodic structure.

Independent direction and Transformation

Dissecting how dynamic cycles impact coordination and how people adjust their activities in light of evolving conditions.

The Close to home Coordination

Feelings are entwined with coordination, affecting our activities and responses in different circumstances. Understanding this close to home aspect is vital for appreciating the coordination association.

Close to home Guideline and Restraint

How close to home guideline and discretion assume crucial parts in keeping up with coordination, especially in high-pressure circumstances.

Social Coordination and Sympathy

Investigating social coordination and sympathy, revealing insight into what our capacity to comprehend others' feelings means for our communications and connections.

Stress, Tension, and Coordination

Analyzing the effect of pressure and tension on coordination, and methodologies for dealing with these profound states to keep up with ideal execution.

The Dance of Social Coordination

Coordination isn't restricted to individual activities; it stretches out to overall vibes and social associations. Understanding social coordination is crucial for powerful cooperation and correspondence.

Nonverbal Correspondence and Non-verbal communication

How nonverbal signs, like non-verbal communication and looks, add to social coordination and convey importance in collaborations.

Collective vibes and Cooperation

The intricacies of overall vibes and cooperation, and how compelling initiative and correspondence are fundamental for fruitful coordination inside gatherings.

Social Varieties in Coordination

Investigating how social standards and practices impact social coordination and the difficulties and potential open doors this presents in different social orders.

Coordination in Regular day to day existence

Coordination is universal, impacting each part of our day to day schedules and cooperations. This section investigates how coordination associates our lives unexpectedly.

Coordination in Medical services

How coordination is basic in medical care settings, from surgeries requiring exact dexterity to the organized endeavors of medical services groups.

Coordination in Schooling

Looking at the job of coordination in schooling, from fine coordinated abilities improvement in youth to the mental coordination expected for critical thinking in advanced education.

Coordination in Artistic expression and Imagination

How coordination becomes the dominant focal point in imaginative pursuits, from dance and theater to painting and figure, and how it fills in as a material for inventive articulation.

Coordination in Sports and Games

The unquestionable association among coordination and sports execution, from group activities to individual undertakings, and the physical and mental coordination expected for greatness.

The Fate of Coordination

As innovation propels and our comprehension of coordination develops, what lies ahead for the coordination association? This part investigates possible future turns of events.

Mechanical Upgrades in Coordination

How arising innovations, like augmented experience and neuroprosthetics, may improve coordination and restore people with coordination-related difficulties.

Coordination in Man-made reasoning

The crossing point of coordination and man-made reasoning, including how computer based intelligence frameworks are being intended to mirror human coordination for different applications.

Coordination in Space Investigation and Mechanical technology

The job of coordination in space investigation and mechanical technology, from independent wanderers on Mars to composed space missions including different nations.

3.1 Defining coordination and its relationship to balance.

Coordination is an idea that penetrates each feature of human existence. It is the ensemble of our muscles, nerves, and cerebrum cooperating to create controlled and intentional developments. Coordination isn't just about actual effortlessness; it reaches out to mental capabilities, close to home guideline, and social associations. One pivotal part of coordination is its natural relationship with balance. In this extensive

investigation, we will analyze the idea of coordination, explain its different aspects, and dig profound into its complicated association with balance.

The Embodiment of Coordination

Before we jump into the connection among coordination and equilibrium, we should begin by characterizing coordination and investigating its complex nature.

Grasping Coordination

Characterizing coordination and analyzing its different parts, including solid coordination, mental coordination, profound coordination, and social coordination.

The Job of the Sensory system

Investigating how the sensory system, containing the focal sensory system (CNS) and the fringe sensory system (PNS), assumes a significant part in organizing different physical processes.

Coordination Across the Life expectancy

Analyzing how coordination creates from outset through youth, immaturity, and into adulthood, featuring the progressions and difficulties each stage brings.

Equilibrium as a Principal Part of Coordination

Balance is a basic piece of coordination. In this part, we will investigate the idea of equilibrium and the way things are complicatedly woven into the texture of coordination.

Characterizing Equilibrium

Characterizing equilibrium and grasping its different parts, including static equilibrium, dynamic equilibrium, and postural control.

The Job of the Vestibular Framework

Digging into the vestibular framework, arranged inside the internal ear, and how it adds to our feeling of equilibrium by identifying changes in head position and development.

Proprioception and Equilibrium

Investigating the job of proprioception, the feeling that permits us to see the position and development of our body parts, in keeping up with balance.

Vision and Equilibrium

Understanding the urgent job of visual contribution to adjust, including how the mind utilizes obvious signals to make changes and redresses to keep up with solidness.

The Neurological Association Among Coordination and Equilibrium

Coordination and equilibrium share a profound neurological association. In this part, we will disentangle the complicated snare of brain processes and signals that underlie this association.

Sensorimotor Coordination

Investigating how the cerebrum coordinates tangible data from the vestibular framework, proprioception, and vision to make an exhaustive image of our body's situation in space.

Engine Control and Equilibrium

Understanding how the mind conveys messages to muscles all through the body, directing changes in muscle tone, stance, and appendage developments to keep up with balance.

The Cerebellum: The Mind's Equilibrium Maestro

Digging into the critical job of the cerebellum, a little yet complex mind locale, in calibrating equilibrium and coordination.

Coordination Difficulties and Equilibrium Problems

Coordination difficulties can appear in different ways, including balance problems. This section investigates normal coordination-related conditions and their effect on balance.

Ataxia: The Disruptor of Equilibrium

Looking at ataxia, a neurological condition portrayed by ungraceful developments and equilibrium issues, and what it means for people's regular routines.

Neurological Issues and Equilibrium

Investigating the connection between neurological issues like Parkinson's infection, numerous sclerosis, and equilibrium hindrances, and examining the board procedures.

Inward Ear Problems and Equilibrium

Understanding how internal ear problems like Meniere's infection and harmless paroxysmal positional dizziness (BPPV) can upset the vestibular framework and lead to adjust issues.

Coordination, Equilibrium, and Active work

Active work and exercise assume a critical part in improving coordination and equilibrium. This part investigates the association between actual wellness and coordination.

Equilibrium Preparing

Investigating different equilibrium preparing practices and their advantages in further developing equilibrium and coordination.

Coordination in Sports and Games

Analyzing how coordination is pivotal for outcome in different games and athletic exercises, from vaulting to hand to hand fighting.

Maturing and Active work

Talking about the significance of active work as people age and how it can assist with keeping up with coordination and equilibrium in later life.

Upgrading Coordination and Equilibrium

Whether for athletic execution, injury anticipation, or regular daily existence, it is vital for upgrade coordination and equilibrium. This part offers down to earth techniques and activities to further develop coordination and equilibrium.

Coordination Activities

A nitty gritty investigation of coordination works out, including proprioceptive drills, dexterity preparing, and dexterity works out.

Equilibrium Improvement Methodologies

Viable tips and procedures to further develop balance, including way of life changes, ecological alterations, and falls anticipation methods.

Coordination in Restoration

How coordination and equilibrium preparing are vital parts of restoration programs for people recuperating from wounds or medical procedures.

Coordination and Equilibrium in Day to day existence

Coordination and equilibrium influence our day to day routines in various ways. This part investigates their importance in ordinary exercises, from preparing a dinner to going across the road.

Coordination in Fine Coordinated movements

How fine coordinated movements, like penmanship and utilizing utensils, grandstand the coordination association in ordinary undertakings.

Equilibrium in Practical Exercises

Looking at how equilibrium assumes a part in exercises like strolling, standing, and exploring different territories.

Mental Coordination in Critical thinking

Understanding how mental coordination and critical thinking abilities are fundamental for ordinary independent direction and performing multiple tasks.

3.2 The neurological basis of coordination.

Coordination is a surprising peculiarity that saturates each part of human existence. From the accuracy of a professional piano player's fingers to the elegant developments of a gymnastic specialist, coordination is the orchestra of our muscles, nerves, and mind working as a unified whole. Understanding the neurological premise of coordination is an excursion into the mind boggling trap of brain processes, signals, and designs that organize these complicated developments. In this investigation, we will dive into the principal neurological cycles that underlie coordination, from the mind's job in arranging and execution to the tactile criticism components that guide everything we might do.

The Cerebrum's Job in Coordination

The cerebrum is the focal center of coordination, where plans are made, signals are sent, and activities are executed. In this part, we will unwind the cerebrum's job in organizing our developments.

The Focal Sensory system

An investigation of the focal sensory system (CNS), comprising of the mind and spinal line, and its essential job in planning both deliberate and compulsory developments.

The Engine Cortex

A profound plunge into the engine cortex, a district of the cerebrum liable for arranging, starting, and controlling deliberate developments. We'll investigate how various pieces of the engine cortex administer explicit body regions.

The Basal Ganglia

Understanding the capability of the basal ganglia, a gathering of cores profound inside the cerebrum, in refining engine developments and choosing fitting activities.

The Cerebellum

Diving into the cerebellum's complicated job in coordination, tweaking developments, and keeping up with equilibrium and stance.

The Neurological Pathways of Coordination

Coordination depends on a tremendous organization of brain connections that send signals from the mind to the muscles. This section investigates the pathways liable for engine control.

The Pyramidal Parcel

Looking at the pyramidal parcel, a significant pathway liable for intentional engine control, and how it communicates signals from the engine cortex to the spinal rope and muscles.

The Extrapyramidal Framework

Investigating the extrapyramidal framework, a complicated organization of brain processes engaged with balancing and directing engine developments, especially those that happen subliminally.

Upper and Lower Engine Neurons

Understanding the job of upper and lower engine neurons in engine control and how their brokenness can prompt coordination issues.

The Coordination Association: Tangible Criticism

Tangible criticism is a basic part of coordination, permitting us to screen our developments and make changes progressively. This part investigates the tactile frameworks that add to coordination.

Proprioception

Investigating proprioception, our natural feeling of where our body parts are in space, and how it adds to coordination by giving ceaseless criticism to the mind.

Vision and Coordination

Figuring out the job of visual criticism in coordination, from following moving items to keeping up with balance and exploring complex conditions.

Vestibular Framework

Diving into the vestibular framework, arranged inside the inward ear, and how it identifies head developments and changes ready, assuming a urgent part in balance and spatial direction.

Somatosensory Framework

Inspecting the somatosensory framework, liable for distinguishing contact, tension, temperature, and agony, and its commitment to coordination and body mindfulness.

Engine Learning and Muscle Memory

Coordination isn't exclusively about executing developments — it likewise includes learning and refining those developments after some time. In this part, we investigate the neurological cycles of engine learning and muscle memory.

The Job of Synaptic Pliancy

Understanding synaptic versatility, the mind's capacity to reinforce or debilitate associations among neurons, and its significance in acquiring and refining coordinated movements.

Muscle Memory

Investigating the idea of muscle memory, where tedious developments lead to changes in the sensory system that upgrade coordination and execution.

The Significance of Training

Featuring the meaning of training and reiteration in engine advancing and how it prompts more proficient coordination.

Coordination Problems and Neurological Difficulties

Neurological difficulties and issues can upset coordination. In this part, we dive into normal coordination issues and their basic neurological systems.

Ataxia

Inspecting ataxia, a neurological problem portrayed by ungraceful developments, and how harm to explicit mind locales or pathways can prompt this condition.

Parkinson's Sickness

Understanding how Parkinson's illness, a neurodegenerative issue, influences coordination and development control, especially because of dopamine lack in the basal ganglia.

Cerebral Paralysis

Investigating cerebral paralysis, a gathering of issues influencing development and stance, and how cerebrum harm during improvement can prompt coordination challenges.

Upgrading Coordination through Neurorehabilitation

Neurorehabilitation is a field committed to further developing coordination and versatility in people with neurological difficulties. This section examines the standards and procedures engaged with neurore-habilitation.

Active recuperation and Recovery

Looking at how active recuperation and recovery programs are customized to people with coordination problems, zeroing in on activities and mediations to improve coordinated abilities.

Word related Treatment

Understanding the job of word related treatment in assisting people with coordination challenges recapture autonomy in everyday exercises.

Assistive Innovations

Investigating how assistive advances, like mind PC interfaces and automated exoskeletons, are being utilized to help coordination and portability in people with neurological circumstances.

The Eventual fate of Neurological Exploration in Coordination

As how we might interpret the neurological premise of coordination extends, additional opportunities and innovations arise. In this last part, we investigate the fate of neurological exploration in coordination.

Cerebrum PC Points of interaction

Examining the capability of cerebrum PC interfaces in upgrading coordination and reestablishing engine capability in people with neurological difficulties.

Brain Pliancy and Recuperation

Analyzing continuous examination into brain versatility and how it might open new roads for restoration and recuperation in coordination problems.

Moral Contemplations

Taking into account the moral ramifications of neurological exploration, especially in regions like mind PC connection points and neuro-enhancement.

Chapter 4

Assessing Your Current State

Surveying your present status is a fundamental stage on the excursion to self-awareness, personal growth, and accomplishing your objectives. It's similar to checking out your life, understanding where you stand, and acquiring clearness about where you need to go. This exhaustive self-assessment guide will assist you with leaving on an excursion of self-disclosure, furnishing you with the instruments and experiences expected to survey your present status across different parts of your life, including your actual wellbeing, mental prosperity, connections, vocation, and self-awareness. Toward the finish of this investigation, you'll have a more clear image of your assets, shortcomings, and regions for development, empowering you to graph a course towards a seriously satisfying and healthy lifestyle.

The Significance of Self-Appraisal

Prior to jumping into the particulars of self-evaluation, we should investigate why it's fundamental and what it can emphatically mean for your life.

The Force of Mindfulness

Understanding the idea of mindfulness and how it shapes the underpinning of self-evaluation and self-awareness.

Advantages of Self-Appraisal

Investigating the various benefits of self-evaluation, from recognizing regions for development to arriving at informed conclusions about your life.

The Association with Objective Setting

Featuring how self-evaluation is unpredictably connected to objective setting, as an unmistakable comprehension of your present status is essential for laying out practical and significant objectives.

Actual Wellbeing Appraisal

Actual wellbeing is the foundation of a satisfying life. This section guides you through surveying your actual prosperity.

Actual Wellness Assessment

Figuring out the parts of actual wellness, including cardiorespiratory perseverance, solid strength, adaptability, and body arrangement, and how to evaluate them.

Nourishment and Diet Investigation

Assessing your dietary propensities, wholesome decisions, and their effect on your general wellbeing and energy levels.

Rest and Rest Evaluation

Surveying the quality and amount of your rest and its effect on your physical and psychological wellness.

Wellbeing Screenings and Clinical Check-Ups

Direction on booking normal wellbeing screenings and check-ups to screen and keep up with your actual wellbeing.

Assessing Your Psychological Prosperity

Mental prosperity is similarly essential for a satisfying life. This part assists you with evaluating your psychological wellness and profound equilibrium.

The ability to appreciate people on a profound level Evaluation

Figuring out capacity to appreciate individuals at their core and evaluating your capacity to perceive, comprehend, and deal with your feelings.

Stress The board Assessment

Investigating your feelings of anxiety, distinguishing stressors, and embracing pressure the board procedures to improve mental prosperity.

Taking care of oneself and Psychological well-being Practices

Evaluating your taking care of oneself schedules and psychological well-being works on, including care, contemplation, and unwinding procedures.

Looking for Proficient Assistance

Perceiving when it's vital for look for proficient help for psychological well-being concerns and decreasing the disgrace encompassing emotional well-being treatment.

Evaluating Your Connections

Solid connections are a foundation of a fantastic life. This part directs you through assessing your connections and social associations.

Family and Individual Connections Evaluation

Evaluating the nature of your associations with relatives, accomplices, and dear companions, and recognizing regions for development.

Group of friends Assessment

Investigating the variety and profundity of your social associations and surveying whether they line up with your qualities and objectives.

Relational abilities Evaluation

Assessing your relational abilities, including undivided attention, sympathy, and compelling articulation, and their effect on your connections.

Compromise and Limits

Evaluating your capacity to explore clashes productively and put down solid stopping points in your connections.

Assessing Your Vocation and Expert Turn of events

Your vocation and expert life assume a critical part in your general prosperity. This part assists you with evaluating your vocation fulfillment and development potential.

Profession Fulfillment Evaluation

Investigating your degree of fulfillment with your present place of employment or vocation way and recognizing factors that add to your expert satisfaction or discontent.

Abilities and Capabilities Examination

Assessing your ongoing range of abilities, recognizing regions for development, and surveying their arrangement with your vocation objectives.

Vocation Development and Improvement Plan

Making an arrangement for your expert development and improvement, including laying out vocation objectives and investigating valuable open doors for progression.

Evaluating Your Self-awareness

Self-improvement is a deep rooted venture. This section guides you through assessing your self-awareness and personal development endeavors.

Individual Objectives and Desires

Evaluating your own objectives, yearnings, and dreams, and analyzing whether your ongoing activities line up with these goals.

Long lasting Mastering and Expertise Improvement

Assessing your obligation to ceaseless mastering and ability improvement, whether through conventional instruction, online courses, or self-study.

Using time effectively and Efficiency

Surveying your time usage abilities, efficiency propensities, and the proficiency of your day to day schedules.

Beating Difficulties and Obstructions

Recognizing and assessing difficulties and deterrents that might be obstructing your self-improvement venture.

Setting Your Appraisal In motion

In this last part, we'll investigate how to utilize the bits of knowledge acquired from your self-evaluation to roll out certain improvements in your day to day existence.

Defining Savvy Objectives

Figuring out how to set Explicit, Quantifiable, Reachable, Significant, and Time-bound (Shrewd) objectives in light of your evaluation discoveries.

Fostering an Activity Plan

Making a bit by bit activity intend to address regions for development and accomplish your objectives.

Checking Progress

Investigating systems for following and assessing your advancement over the long run to guarantee you stay on the way to personal development.

Looking for Help and Responsibility

Figuring out the benefit of looking for help from tutors, mentors, or responsibility accomplices to assist you with accomplishing your objectives.

4.1Self-assessment tools and tests for balance and coordination.

Equilibrium and coordination are basic parts of human development and are basic for performing different exercises of day to day living, sports, and keeping up with generally speaking wellbeing. Impeded equilibrium and coordination can prompt falls, wounds, and diminished personal satisfaction. To survey and work on these capacities, different self-evaluation apparatuses and tests have been created. This thorough aide investigates the significance of equilibrium and coordination, the variables influencing

them, and a point by point assessment of self-evaluation instruments and tests accessible for people to assess and upgrade their equilibrium and coordination.

Presentation

Equilibrium and coordination are mind boggling neuromuscular abilities that include the reconciliation of tactile data, engine control, and proprioception. These capacities are fundamental for keeping up with strength, controlling development, and performing undertakings with accuracy and productivity. Balance alludes to the capacity to keep an upstanding stance and harmony, while coordination includes the amicable execution of coordinated movements.

Significance of Equilibrium and Coordination:

Fall Counteraction: Equilibrium and coordination assume a vital part in forestalling falls, particularly in more established grown-ups. Falls can prompt extreme wounds, decreased freedom, and expanded medical services costs.

Athletic Execution: Competitors, no matter what their game, depend on equilibrium and coordination for spryness, speed, and exactness. Further developed equilibrium and coordination can upgrade sports execution and lessen the gamble of injury.

Useful Freedom: Fundamental everyday exercises like strolling, climbing steps, and going after objects require sufficient equilibrium and coordination. Hindrances in these abilities can frustrate free living.

Recovery: People recuperating from wounds or medical procedures frequently need to recapture their equilibrium and coordination to securely get back to their typical exercises.

By and large Wellbeing: Great equilibrium and coordination add to generally wellbeing and prosperity, as they permit people to participate in proactive tasks that advance cardiovascular wellness and muscle strength.

Factors Influencing Equilibrium and Coordination

1. **Age:** Equilibrium and coordination will more often than not decline with age because of changes in muscle strength, joint adaptability, and tangible discernment.
2. **Neurological Circumstances:** Conditions like various sclerosis, Parkinson's sickness, and stroke can debilitate the focal sensory system's capacity to control equilibrium and coordination.
3. **Solid Strength and Perseverance:** Feeble muscles, particularly those in the center and lower appendages, can think twice about and coordination.

4. **Tangible Capability:** Weakened vision, hearing, or proprioception can disturb the tactile information fundamental for keeping up with balance.

5. **Prescriptions:** Certain meds might influence a singular's equilibrium and coordination as an incidental effect.

6. **Vestibular Framework Problems:** Issues of the inward ear's vestibular framework can prompt unsteadiness and awkwardness.

7. **Mental Elements:** Nervousness and stress can impact coordination and equilibrium through their effect on muscle pressure and concentration.

Self-Appraisal Apparatuses and Tests for Equilibrium and Coordination

1. **Berg Equilibrium Scale (BBS)**

   Reason: The BBS is broadly used to evaluate balance in more seasoned grown-ups and people with neurological circumstances. It comprises of 14 errands that assess static and dynamic equilibrium.

   Scoring: The test is scored on a scale from 0 to 56, with higher scores demonstrating better equilibrium. Scores under 45 are characteristic of an expanded fall risk.

   Methodology: People perform undertakings like remaining on one foot, going after objects, and changing situations while being scored in view of their presentation.

   Benefits: The BBS is a solid and approved device with laid out standards for different populaces.

   Limits: It may not be reasonable for people with extreme versatility disabilities.

2. **Coordinated Up and Go Test (Pull)**

   Reason: The Pull surveys utilitarian portability and is normally utilized in clinical settings to anticipate fall risk.

   System: The singular beginnings in a situated position, stands up, strolls three meters, turns, returns, and puts down. The time taken to finish the job is recorded.

Translation: Longer times show expanded fall risk, with explicit shorts characterizing different gamble levels.

Benefits: The Pull is easy to manage and requires insignificant hardware.

Restrictions: It may not catch unobtrusive equilibrium deficiencies.

3. **Utilitarian Arrive at Test (FRT)**

   Reason: The FRT estimates a singular's capacity to reach forward while keeping up with balance, making it a dependable mark of dynamic equilibrium.

   Technique: The singular stands close to a wall with an arm broadened, and the distance they can reach forward without losing balance is estimated.

   Understanding: More noteworthy arrive at distances connote better unique equilibrium.

   Benefits: The FRT is not difficult to perform and requires negligible hardware.

   Limits: It fundamentally surveys forward balance control.

4. **Single Leg Position Test**

   Reason: This test assesses a singular's capacity to adjust on one leg and is frequently used to recognize impedances in proprioception and lower appendage strength.

   Method: The singular stands on one leg with their eyes open as far as might be feasible. The test can be rehashed with eyes shut.

   Understanding: Longer terms demonstrate better equilibrium and proprioception.

   Benefits: a straightforward test should be possible anyplace without extraordinary gear.

   Constraints: It may not give a far reaching evaluation of equilibrium.

5. **Romberg Test**

   Reason: The Romberg test surveys a singular's capacity to keep up with offset with their eyes shut, principally assessing proprioception.

   Method: The individual stands with their feet together, arms at their sides, and eyes shut. The evaluator notices for influencing or loss of equilibrium.

   Understanding: Influencing or loss of equilibrium might show proprioceptive deficiencies.

   Benefits: It's not difficult to oversee and requires negligible hardware.

   Constraints: It centers basically around proprioception and may not recognize other equilibrium issues.

6. **Small scale Absolute best (Little Equilibrium Assessment Frameworks Test)**

   Reason: The Smaller than expected Absolute best is an abbreviated rendition of the Absolute best, intended to survey offset in people with neurological circumstances.

   Methodology: It incorporates 14 things that assess different parts of equilibrium, including expectant, responsive, and tangible parts.

   Understanding: The test gives an all out score, with lower scores showing more prominent equilibrium disability.

   Benefits: It offers a complete evaluation of offset in people with neurological circumstances.

   Constraints: Longer organization time contrasted with a few different tests.

7. **Y-Equilibrium Test (YBT)**

   Reason: The Y-Equilibrium Test surveys dynamic equilibrium and useful security by estimating the arrive at distance in three headings.

   Methodology: The singular stands on one leg and spans beyond what many would consider possible in three headings (front, posteromedial, and posterolateral) utilizing the other leg.

Understanding: More noteworthy arrive at distances are related with better powerful equilibrium and diminished injury risk.

Benefits: It gives a utilitarian evaluation of equilibrium and can be utilized in sports settings.

Impediments: Requires specific gear (Y-Equilibrium Unit).

8. **Dynamic Step List (DGI)**

Reason: The DGI surveys a singular's capacity to alter their step design in light of various errands, like strolling at various velocities or turning.

Technique: It comprises of eight undertakings, and people are scored in view of their presentation.

Translation: Lower scores demonstrate step and equilibrium issues.

Benefits: Gives experiences into dynamic equilibrium during stride.

Impediments: May not be reasonable for people with extreme portability hindrances.

9. **Adjusted Falls Viability Scale (MFES)**

Reason: The MFES surveys a singular's trust in their capacity to perform different exercises without falling.

Methodology: People rate their certainty on a scale for every movement recorded, like strolling on frosty walkways or ascending a stepping stool.

Understanding: Lower scores demonstrate lower trust in equilibrium and coordination capacities.

Benefits: Valuable for surveying the mental part of equilibrium.

Limits: May not straightforwardly measure actual equilibrium and coordination.

10. **NeuroCom Equilibrium Expert Framework**

Reason: This exceptional framework surveys equilibrium and coordination utilizing modernized dynamic posturography, giving point by point information on a singular's equilibrium execution.

Strategy: The singular stands on a stage that actions postural influence during different errands, like remaining on one leg or keeping up with balance on a temperamental surface.

Translation: The framework gives objective information on balance execution.

Benefits: Offers exact evaluation and is frequently utilized in clinical and research settings.

Impediments: Requires particular gear and prepared faculty.

4.2 Identifying areas that need improvement.

Recognizing regions that need improvement is a basic part of individual and expert development. Whether you are a singular looking for personal growth or a business intending to improve its tasks, pinpointing regions for improvement is the most important move towards accomplishing positive change. In this exhaustive aide, we will investigate the significance of perceiving regions that require improvement, the techniques and apparatuses accessible for evaluation, and systems for actually addressing these regions to cultivate development and achievement.

Presentation

Improvement is a consistent cycle in both individual and expert circles of life. It is driven by the acknowledgment that there are regions in which we can improve, be it in our abilities, information, propensities, or frameworks and cycles. Distinguishing these regions is the establishment whereupon significant advancement is constructed. Without a reasonable comprehension of what needs improvement, it is trying to define objectives, foster techniques, or measure achievement.

The Significance of Recognizing Regions for Development

Upgraded Execution: Perceiving and addressing shortcomings or lacks can prompt better execution, whether in the work environment, sports, or individual life.

Upper hand: In the business world, recognizing regions that need improvement can give a strategic advantage by smoothing out tasks, expanding productivity, and conveying better items or administrations.

Self-awareness: On a singular level, recognizing regions that require improvement is fundamental for self-improvement and self-advancement.

Compromise: Distinguishing areas of progress can help in settling clashes, whether in connections, groups, or associations, by resolving basic issues.

Transformation to Change: In a quickly impacting world, perceiving regions for development considers flexibility and strength notwithstanding new difficulties and open doors.

Techniques and Instruments for Distinguishing Regions That Need Improvement

There are different techniques and apparatuses accessible to assist people and associations with distinguishing regions that require improvement. These methodologies can be custom fitted to explicit settings and targets. Here are a few generally utilized strategies:

1. **Self-Appraisal**
   Reason: Self-appraisal includes contemplation and self-reflection to distinguish individual regions that need improvement. It is a significant instrument for self-improvement.
   Process:
   Put away devoted time for reflection.
   Recognize your assets and shortcomings.
   Look for input from confided in companions, family, or associates.
   Utilize self-evaluation apparatuses and surveys intended for explicit areas of progress.
   Benefits: Self-evaluation is a savvy and available strategy, giving profound experiences into self-awareness potential open doors.

Constraints: It could be one-sided or restricted by one's self-discernment.

2. **360-Degree Input**

Reason: 360-degree criticism gathers input from numerous sources, including peers, bosses, subordinates, and self-evaluation, to give an all encompassing perspective on a singular's assets and regions for development.

Process:

Unknown studies are directed, requesting that members assess the singular's exhibition and conduct.

The input is accumulated and imparted to the individual, advancing mindfulness.

Benefits: 360-degree input offers a balanced viewpoint and can reveal vulnerable sides.

Impediments: It could be impacted by predisposition or political variables, and namelessness can once in a while prompt unconstructive remarks.

3. **SWOT Investigation (Qualities, Shortcomings, Open doors, Dangers)**

Reason: SWOT investigation is an essential arranging device utilized by organizations to distinguish inside qualities and shortcomings and outside potential open doors and dangers.

Process:

List inward qualities and shortcomings, like abilities, assets, and cycles.

Recognize outside open doors and dangers, for example, market patterns, contest, and monetary elements.

Break down the connections between these elements to decide regions for development.

Benefits: SWOT examination gives an organized way to deal with recognizing improvement regions inside a hierarchical setting.

Constraints: It may not give nitty gritty bits of knowledge into individual execution or self-awareness.

4. **Key Execution Pointers (KPIs)**

   Reason: KPIs are quantifiable measurements that action the presentation of people, groups, or associations. Recognizing regions for development can be founded on KPI examination.

   Process:

   Characterize important KPIs in view of authoritative objectives.

   Consistently evaluate execution against these KPIs.

   Distinguish regions where execution misses the mark concerning targets.

   Benefits: KPIs offer an information driven way to deal with pinpointing improvement regions and following advancement.

   Limits: KPIs may not catch all parts of execution or individual development.

5. **Underlying driver Examination**

   Reason: Main driver examination plans to recognize the basic reasons for issues or difficulties, assisting with pinpointing regions in cycles or frameworks that require improvement.

   Process:

   Recognize a particular issue or issue.

   Examine the causes utilizing devices like the "5 Whys" or Fishbone Graph (Ishikawa outline).

   Decide the root cause(s) and foster answers for address them.

   Benefits: Underlying driver investigation helps address foundational issues and further develop processes.

   Impediments: It tends to be tedious, and the investigation may not uncover every contributing component.

6. **Benchmarking**

   Reason: Benchmarking includes contrasting an association's presentation or practices against industry principles or contenders to distinguish regions where it lingers behind.

   Process:

   Recognize key execution regions for examination.

Accumulate information on contenders or industry pioneers in those areas.

Examine the holes and focus on regions for development.

Benefits: Benchmarking gives a cutthroat viewpoint and sets clear execution targets.

Restrictions: It may not think about one of a kind conditions or factors that influence execution.

Procedures for Tending to Regions That Need Improvement

Recognizing regions that need improvement is only the initial step. Successfully tending to these areas requires smart methodologies and activities. Here are techniques that people and associations can utilize:

1. **Put forth Clear Objectives**

   Characterize explicit, quantifiable, attainable, pertinent, and time-bound (Shrewd) objectives for development. Clear objectives give guidance and inspiration.

2. **Focus on Progress Regions**

   Not all regions requiring improvement are similarly basic. Focus on them in view of their effect and attainability. Center around high-need regions first.

3. **Foster Activity Plans**

   Make point by point activity plans framing the means expected for development. These plans ought to incorporate achievements and cutoff times.

4. **Look for Preparing and Training**

   Put resources into preparing, courses, studios, or instructing to foster the abilities and information fundamental for development.

5. **Execute Input Circles**

   Lay out systems for continuous input and assessment to follow progress and change procedures depending on the situation.

6. **Embrace Persistent Learning**

   Develop a culture of persistent learning and improvement inside associations and in self-improvement. Energize interest and versatility.

7. **Work together and Look for Help**
Team up with partners, tutors, or mentors who can give direction and backing in areas of progress.

8. **Measure and Assess Progress**
Routinely survey and measure progress utilizing pertinent measurements, KPIs, or appraisals. Change procedures in light of results.

9. **Observe Accomplishments**
Recognize and commend accomplishments and achievements along the way of progress to keep up with inspiration and force.

10. **Emphasize and Refine Procedures**

Perceive that improvement is a continuous cycle. Persistently refine systems and adjust to changing conditions and objectives.

Chapter 5

Enhancing Balance

Balance is an essential part of human capability that influences virtually every feature of our lives, from fundamental day to day exercises like strolling to additional mind boggling undertakings like athletic execution. Whether you're an expert competitor hoping to acquire an upper hand, a more seasoned grown-up trying to diminish the gamble of falls, or basically somebody keen on further developing their general prosperity, improving equilibrium is an objective that can help everybody. In this far reaching guide, we will investigate the idea of equilibrium, its importance, the elements that impact it, and various procedures, activities, and methods to assist people of any age and capacities with upgrading their equilibrium.

1. **Prologue to Adjust**
   Figuring out Equilibrium
   Balance is a central part of human usefulness that frequently slips through the cracks until it becomes compromised. It includes the capacity to keep up with harmony, soundness, and command over one's body in different positions and during various developments. Accomplishing and keeping up with balance requires

multifaceted coordination among different frameworks in the body, including the outer muscle, tactile, and sensory systems.

Adjusting includes a few key parts:

Tactile Info: The body depends on tangible data from different sources to grasp its situation in space. This incorporates input from the visual framework (eyes), the vestibular framework (internal ear), and proprioception (familiarity with body position and development).

Focal Sensory system: The cerebrum processes tangible information and conveys messages to the muscles to change act and keep up with balance. It ceaselessly refreshes these signs in light of evolving conditions.

Outer muscle Framework: Muscles assume a urgent part in keeping up with balance. They give the fundamental strength and coordination to balance out the body during developments.

Adjusting happens in a great many exercises, from straightforward behaves like standing and strolling to additional complicated developments like moving, playing sports, or performing gymnastics. A powerful interaction adjusts to different circumstances and conditions.

Why Equilibrium Matters

Balance isn't just about keeping away from falls; it has sweeping ramifications for by and large wellbeing, prosperity, and personal satisfaction. The following are a few motivations behind why equilibrium is critical:

Fall Counteraction: Keeping up with balance is critical for forestalling falls, particularly among more established grown-ups. Falls can bring about serious wounds, decreased versatility, and a deficiency of freedom.

Athletic Execution: Competitors depend on balance for dexterity, coordination, and injury avoidance. Upgrading equilibrium can further develop sports execution and lessen the gamble of sports-related wounds.

Useful Autonomy: Regular exercises, for example, getting up, climbing steps, and going after objects require great equilibrium. Weakened equilibrium can block free living.

Recovery: Individuals recuperating from wounds or medical procedures frequently need to recapture their equilibrium to get back to their typical exercises securely.

Generally Wellbeing: Great equilibrium adds to by and large wellbeing by empowering proactive tasks that advance cardio-vascular wellness, muscle strength, and adaptability.

Personal satisfaction: A solid feeling of equilibrium upgrades one's capacity to take part in relaxation exercises, travel, and take part in get-togethers with certainty.

As we age, balance will in general decay because of different age-related changes, for example, diminished bulk and strength, diminished joint adaptability, and adjusted tactile discernment. Be that as it may, balance not set in stone by age, and people, all things considered, can profit from balance-upgrading techniques.

2. **Factors Influencing Equilibrium**

A few variables can impact a singular's equilibrium. Understanding these variables is fundamental for tending to adjust issues successfully. Here are a few key factors that can influence balance:

Age

Decreased Bulk and Strength: Maturing is related with a characteristic loss of bulk and strength, especially in the lower appendages, which are significant for keeping up with balance.

Diminished Joint Adaptability: Solidifying of the joints, especially in the hips, knees, and lower legs, can influence a singular's capacity to change their situation and keep up with steadiness.

Modified Tactile Discernment: Age-related changes in the visual, vestibular (inward ear), and proprioceptive frameworks can prompt decreased tangible info, making it more testing to see changes ready and answer likewise.

More slow Reflexes: Maturing can dial back reflexes and response times, which are fundamental for making fast acclimations to keep up with balance.

This multitude of changes can add to an expanded gamble of falls in more seasoned grown-ups.

Solid Strength and Perseverance

Solid strength and perseverance assume a basic part in balance. Feeble muscles, particularly in the center, hips, and lower appendages, can think twice about and coordination. Interestingly, people areas of strength for with are better prepared to control their developments and keep up with balance.

Tangible Capability

Visual Framework: The eyes give urgent data about the climate and assist people with situating themselves. Disabled vision, whether because of eye conditions or unfortunate lighting, can influence balance.

Vestibular Framework: The internal ear contains the vestibular framework, which recognizes changes in head position and development. Problems or conditions influencing the vestibular framework can disturb balance.

Proprioception: Proprioception alludes to the body's attention to its situation in space. It depends on criticism from tangible receptors in the muscles and joints. Proprioceptive shortfalls can prompt equilibrium issues.

Neurological Circumstances

Certain neurological circumstances can weaken the focal sensory system's capacity to control equilibrium and coordination. Conditions like various sclerosis, Parkinson's illness, and stroke can influence equilibrium and increment the gamble of falls.

Drugs

A few drugs, including tranquilizers, antihypertensives, and anti-depressants, can cause unsteadiness or influence a singular's equilibrium. It's fundamental to know about possible secondary effects and examine them with a medical services supplier.

Mental Variables

Mental elements like uneasiness and stress can impact coordination and equilibrium through their effect on muscle pressure and concentration. People encountering elevated degrees of stress or tension might observe that their equilibrium is briefly compromised.

It's critical to take note of that numerous people might encounter a mix of these elements, making it vital for address them extensively while dealing with balance upgrade.

3. Surveying Your Equilibrium

Surveying your ongoing equilibrium level is an essential initial phase in the excursion to improving equilibrium. Self-evaluation instruments and tests can give important bits of knowledge into your equilibrium capacities. Also, medical care experts can lead more extensive appraisals. We should investigate a few normal techniques for evaluating balance:

Self-Appraisal Instruments and Tests

1. **Berg Equilibrium Scale (BBS)**

    Reason: The BBS is generally used to evaluate balance, particularly in more seasoned grown-ups and people with neurological circumstances. It comprises of 14 errands that assess both static and dynamic equilibrium.

    Scoring: The test is scored on a scale from 0 to 56, with higher scores showing better equilibrium. Scores under 45 are characteristic of an expanded fall risk.

    Strategy: People perform undertakings like remaining on one foot, going after objects, and changing situations while being scored in view of their exhibition.

    Benefits: The BBS is a dependable and approved instrument with laid out standards for different populaces.

    Impediments: It may not be appropriate for people with extreme versatility debilitations.

2. **Planned Up and Go Test (Pull)**

   Reason: The Pull evaluates practical portability and is usually utilized in clinical settings to anticipate fall risk.

   Methodology: It includes the singular beginning in a situated position, standing up, strolling three meters, turning, returning, and putting down. The time taken to finish the job is recorded.

   Translation: Longer times show expanded fall risk, with explicit shorts characterizing different gamble levels.

   Benefits: The Pull is easy to regulate and requires insignificant hardware.

   Impediments: It may not catch unpretentious equilibrium shortfalls.

3. **Useful Arrive at Test (FRT)**

   Reason: The FRT estimates a singular's capacity to reach forward while keeping up with balance, making it a solid mark of dynamic equilibrium.

   Methodology: The singular stands close to a wall with an arm broadened, and the distance they can reach forward without losing balance is estimated.

   Understanding: More noteworthy arrive at distances connote better powerful equilibrium.

   Benefits: The FRT is not difficult to perform and requires insignificant hardware.

   Constraints: It principally evaluates forward balance control.

4. **Single Leg Position Test**

   Reason: This test assesses a singular's capacity to adjust on one leg and is frequently used to distinguish disabilities in proprioception and lower appendage strength.

   Technique: The singular stands on one leg with their eyes open as far as might be feasible. The test can be rehashed with eyes shut.

   Understanding: Longer terms demonstrate better equilibrium and proprioception.

Benefits: a straightforward test should be possible anyplace without exceptional hardware.

Limits: It may not give an exhaustive evaluation of equilibrium.

5. **Romberg Test**

Reason: The Romberg test surveys a singular's capacity to keep up with offset with their eyes shut, principally assessing proprioception.

Method: The individual stands with their feet together, arms at their sides, and eyes shut. The evaluator notices for influencing or loss of equilibrium.

Understanding: Influencing or loss of equilibrium might demonstrate proprioceptive shortfalls.

Benefits: It's not difficult to oversee and requires insignificant hardware.

Constraints: It centers fundamentally around proprioception and may not distinguish other equilibrium issues.

6. **Small scale Absolute best (Little Equilibrium Assessment Frameworks Test)**

Reason: The Small scale Absolute best is an abbreviated variant of the Absolute best, intended to evaluate offset in people with neurological circumstances.

System: It incorporates 14 things that assess different parts of equilibrium, including expectant, receptive, and tactile parts.

Understanding: The test gives a complete score, with lower scores demonstrating more noteworthy equilibrium impedance.

Benefits: It offers an exhaustive evaluation of offset in people with neurological circumstances.

Restrictions: Longer organization time contrasted with a few different tests.

7. **Y-Equilibrium Test (YBT)**

Reason: The Y-Equilibrium Test surveys dynamic equilibrium and utilitarian dependability by estimating the arrive at distance in three headings.

Method: The singular stands on one leg and compasses beyond what many would consider possible in three headings (foremost, posteromedial, and posterolateral) utilizing the other leg.

Translation: More noteworthy arrive at distances are related with better powerful equilibrium and diminished injury risk.

Benefits: It gives a utilitarian evaluation of equilibrium and can be utilized in sports settings.

Restrictions: Requires specific hardware (Y-Equilibrium Pack).

8. **Dynamic Step File (DGI)**

Reason: The DGI surveys a singular's capacity to adjust their stride design in light of various errands, like strolling at various velocities or turning.

Technique: It comprises of eight undertakings, and people are scored in view of their exhibition.

Understanding: Lower scores show stride and equilibrium issues.

Benefits: Gives bits of knowledge into dynamic equilibrium during stride.

Restrictions: May not be appropriate for people with extreme portability disabilities.

Proficient Evaluation

While self-appraisal devices and tests are important for acquiring experiences into your equilibrium, talking with medical care experts is urgent, particularly on the off chance that you have existing ailments or worries about your equilibrium. Medical services experts, like actual specialists, word related advisors, and vestibular advisors, can direct

far reaching evaluations, recognize hidden issues, and foster customized balance improvement plans.

Actual specialists, specifically, assume a critical part in assessing and further developing equilibrium. They might utilize particular hardware, for example, force plates and electronic dynamic posturography frameworks, to dispassionately survey balance more. Moreover, they can configuration fitted activity programs and give involved direction to address explicit equilibrium deficiencies.

4. Methodologies for Improving Equilibrium

Whenever you've evaluated your equilibrium and recognized regions that need improvement, now is the ideal time to carry out systems to upgrade your equilibrium. These techniques incorporate a scope of activities, way of life changes, and contemplations for different populaces.

Strength Preparing

Strong strength and perseverance are necessary parts of equilibrium. Strength preparing works out, especially those focusing on the center, hips, and lower appendages, can assist with further developing equilibrium by improving the security of the body's establishment.

Works out:

Squats

Lurches

Boards

Leg raises

Hip scaffolds

Proprioception Activities

Proprioception practices challenge and work on the body's familiarity with its situation in space, a critical calculate balance upgrade.

Works out:

Balance on lopsided surfaces (froth cushions, balance sheets)

Single-leg balance works out

Eyes-shut balance drills

Remaining on one foot with fluctuated arm developments

Yoga and Jujitsu

Yoga and Jujitsu are antiquated practices that advance equilibrium, adaptability, and body mindfulness. Standard support in these disciplines can altogether further develop equilibrium and by and large prosperity.

Benefits:

Further developed adaptability

Improved body mindfulness

Stress decrease

Better stance

Balance Gear and Devices

Different equilibrium upgrading instruments and gear are accessible, going from strength balls and equilibrium sheets to froth rollers and wobble pads. Consolidating these into your wellness routine can challenge your equilibrium in powerful ways.

Useful Preparation

Useful preparation emulates genuine developments and difficulties balance in reasonable settings. It is especially significant for competitors and people seeking work on their equilibrium for explicit exercises.

Works out:

Box hops

Medication ball works out

Dexterity stepping stool drills

Sport-explicit equilibrium drills

Center Fortifying

The center assumes a focal part in equilibrium and strength. Center reinforcing activities can assist with keeping an upstanding stance and forestall falls.

Works out:

Boards

Russian turns

Bike crunches

Superman works out

Nourishment and Hydration

Nourishment can affect balance in a roundabout way by impacting factors like muscle wellbeing, bone thickness, and generally speaking prosperity. Guarantee your eating routine gives fundamental supplements to keeping up with actual wellbeing.

Contemplations:

Adequate protein consumption for muscle upkeep and fix.

Satisfactory calcium and vitamin D for bone wellbeing.

Legitimate hydration to forestall dazedness and parchedness related balance issues.

Rest and Stress The executives

Sufficient rest and stress the board are fundamental parts of equilibrium upgrade. Absence of rest and constant pressure can impede mental capability and coordination, adversely influencing balance.

Tips:

Go for the gold long stretches of value rest each evening.

Practice pressure decrease methods like contemplation, profound breathing, and care.

Natural Contemplations

Simplifying alterations to your living and workplaces can add to all the more likely equilibrium and decrease the gamble of falls.

Tips:

Continue to live spaces sufficiently bright.

Eliminate trip dangers and mess from walkways.

Introduce handrails in flights of stairs and restrooms.

Wear suitable footwear with great foothold.

5. Balance Upgrade for Explicit Populaces

Adjusting activities and systems can be customized to explicit populaces to address their exceptional necessities and objectives. Here are a few contemplations for improving equilibrium in unambiguous gatherings:

More established Grown-ups

Improving equilibrium in more established grown-ups is significant for fall counteraction and keeping up with autonomy. Activities ought to zero in on further developing leg strength, adaptability, and proprioception. Kendo and Yoga are superb choices for more established grown-ups.

Competitors

Competitors require explicit equilibrium preparing to succeed in their picked sports and lessen the gamble of injury. Sports-explicit penetrates and activities ought to be coordinated into their preparation regimens.

People with Neurological Circumstances

Individuals with conditions like Parkinson's illness or various sclerosis might encounter balance hindrances. Designated practices and non-intrusive treatment can assist with further developing equilibrium and coordination while overseeing explicit side effects.

Kids and Teenagers

Adjusting activities can help kids and teenagers by advancing engine expertise advancement and diminishing the gamble of wounds during proactive tasks and sports.

6. Forestalling Falls

Falls are a huge concern, particularly for more established grown-ups. Forestalling falls is a basic part of equilibrium improvement. We should investigate a few techniques for fall counteraction:

Fall Chance Evaluation

Lead a complete fall risk evaluation, either freely or with the assistance of medical care experts. This evaluation ought to consider factors like age, clinical history, drugs, and home climate.

Fall Avoidance Methodologies

Carry out fall counteraction techniques in light of the recognized gamble factors. These may incorporate activity programs, vision remedy, prescription changes, and home alterations.

Home Security Measures

Make fundamental adjustments to the home climate to decrease fall risk. Introduce handrails, eliminate free carpets, further develop lighting, and guarantee that generally utilized things are inside simple reach.

7. Proficient Direction and Restoration

In instances of extreme equilibrium issues, complex ailments, or recovery needs, it's essential to look for proficient direction and restoration administrations. Here are a few choices:

Non-intrusive treatment

Actual specialists are specialists in evaluating and further developing equilibrium. They can make customized practice programs, utilize specific gear, and give involved direction to improve balance and forestall falls.

Word related Treatment

Word related advisors center around working on a singular's capacity to perform day to day exercises, including those that require balance. They can suggest assistive gadgets, show versatile procedures, and alter the home climate for better equilibrium.

Vestibular Recovery

People with vestibular problems influencing the internal ear's equilibrium framework might profit from vestibular restoration. This particular treatment plans to retrain the cerebrum to adjust to the issue and further develop balance.

5.1Physical exercises and training techniques for better balance.

Balance is a crucial part of human development and usefulness. It assumes a significant part in our regular routines, from straightforward errands like standing and strolling to additional perplexing exercises like games and moving. Keeping up with great equilibrium is fundamental for forestalling falls and wounds, particularly as we age. Luckily, equilibrium can be improved and kept up with through different actual activities and preparing procedures.

This far reaching guide will investigate the significance of equilibrium, the elements that influence it, and many activities and preparing strategies intended to upgrade balance. Whether you're a competitor hoping to further develop execution or a more established grown-up expecting to forestall falls, these strategies can help people of any age and wellness levels.

The Significance of Equilibrium

Balance is the capacity to keep up with harmony and strength while performing different developments and exercises. It includes the coordination of tactile contribution from the visual, vestibular (inward ear), and proprioceptive (muscle and joint) frameworks. Great equilibrium is essential in light of multiple factors:

Fall Counteraction: Falls are a main source of injury, particularly among more seasoned grown-ups. Solid equilibrium can assist with diminishing the gamble of falls and their related wounds.

Worked on Athletic Execution: Equilibrium is a basic part of many games and proactive tasks, like vaulting, yoga, and hand to hand fighting. Competitors with better equilibrium frequently perform at a more significant level.

Utilitarian Autonomy: Keeping up with balance is fundamental for ordinary undertakings like getting up, strolling, and climbing steps. It adds to generally utilitarian autonomy.

Injury Counteraction: Better equilibrium can lessen the gamble of wounds in exercises that require readiness, for example, trail running or skiing.

Factors Influencing Equilibrium

Age: Offset will in general downfall with age because of changes in muscle strength, joint adaptability, and tangible discernment.

Muscle Strength: Powerless muscles, particularly those in the legs and center, can hinder balance.

Proprioception: The body's attention to its situation in space depends on proprioceptive information. Conditions that influence proprioception, like neuropathy, can affect balance.

Internal Ear Capability: The inward ear assumes a basic part in balance. Conditions influencing the vestibular framework can prompt equilibrium issues.

Visual Information: Vision gives significant prompts to adjust. Visual debilitations or aggravations can influence balance.

Neurological Circumstances: Conditions like Parkinson's illness, various sclerosis, or stroke can disturb balance.

Drugs: Certain prescriptions can have incidental effects that effect equilibrium and coordination.

Natural Elements: Lopsided landscape, unfortunate lighting, and hindrances in the climate can challenge balance.

Now that we've laid out the meaning of equilibrium and the variables that impact it, how about we investigate different actual activities and preparing procedures to improve and keep up with balance.

Activities and Preparing Strategies for Better Equilibrium
Static Equilibrium Activities:

1. **Single-leg Equilibrium:** Stand on one foot with the other foot took off the ground. Stand firm on the footing for 30 seconds to a moment, then, at that point, switch legs.
2. **Couple Position:** Spot one foot straightforwardly before the other and stand firm on the foothold for 30 seconds to a moment. This exercise difficulties your equilibrium by decreasing your base of help.
3. **Tree Posture (Yoga):** Stand on one leg and spot the underside of your other foot on your inward thigh or calf. Center around a direct before you toward further develop equilibrium and hold for 30 seconds to a moment.

Dynamic Equilibrium Activities:

1. **Impact point to-Toe Walk:** Stroll in an orderly fashion by setting the impact point of one foot straightforwardly before the toes of the other. This exercise mirrors the pair position while moving.
2. **Side Leg Raises:** Stand close to a seat or wall for help, then lift one leg out to the side while keeping up with balance on the other. This exercise reinforces the hip abductors, which are critical for balance.
3. **Clock Reach:** Envision remaining in the focal point of a clock. Reach forward to 12 o'clock, then, at that point, to 3 o'clock, 6 o'clock, and 9 o'clock, all while adjusting on one leg. Rehash on the other leg.

Balance Preparing Hardware:

1. **Balance Sheets:** These sheets have a temperamental surface that challenges your equilibrium. You can perform different activities while remaining on them, like squats or turns.
2. **Bosu Balls:** A Bosu ball is a half-vault stage that can be utilized with the level side down or up. It's magnificent for balance preparing and can be utilized for practices like squats, lurches, and boards.
3. **Steadiness Balls:** These huge inflatable balls are flexible devices for balance preparing. You can perform practices like situated leg lifts or steadiness ball spans.

Yoga and Kendo:

1. **Yoga:** Yoga consolidates represents that challenge equilibrium, adaptability, and strength. Rehearses like Hatha or Vinyasa yoga can altogether work on by and large equilibrium.
2. **Jujitsu:** Kendo is a Chinese military craftsmanship known for its sluggish, streaming developments. It improves equilibrium, coordination, and care.

Strength Preparing:

1. **Leg Strength:** Activities like squats, lurches, and calf raises can further develop leg strength, which is critical for balance.
2. **Center Strength:** A solid center settles the middle and upgrades by and large equilibrium. Boards, Russian turns, and supermans are compelling center activities.

Deftness Preparing:

1. **Deftness Stepping stool Penetrates:** These drills include quick and exact footwork through stepping stool like examples on the ground. They further develop coordination and equilibrium.
2. **Cone Drills:** Set up cones in different examples and work on zigzagging all around them rapidly. This mirrors the dexterity required in sports like soccer and b-ball.

Proprioception Preparing:

1. **Balance Cushion Activities:** Utilizing a froth balance cushion, perform practices like remaining on one leg or doing squats. The unsteady surface difficulties proprioception.
2. **Balance Games:** Computer games or applications intended for balance preparing, like the Nintendo Wii Fit, can be fun ways of further developing proprioception.

Vision Upgrade:

1. **Eye-Following Activities:** Work on following articles with your eyes without moving your head. This can upgrade your visual contribution for balance.
2. **Vision-Animating Equilibrium Activities:** Perform offset practices with your eyes shut to depend more on proprioception and internal ear input.

Care and Contemplation:

1. **Care:** Care practices can further develop concentration and focus, which are fundamental for keeping up with balance.
2. **Contemplation:** Reflection methods like body examine contemplation can build consciousness of substantial sensations and further develop proprioception.

Moderate Preparation Plans:

1. **Slow Movement:** Begin with fundamental equilibrium practices and continuously make them more testing as you get to the next level.
2. **Organized Projects:** Consider joining an equilibrium explicit class or program drove by a certified educator to guarantee protected and compelling preparation.

5.2 Lifestyle adjustments and nutritional considerations.

Carrying on with a solid existence isn't simply the shortfall of sickness however a condition of physical, mental, and social prosperity. Accomplishing this equilibrium requires a mix of way of life changes and healthful contemplations. In this complete aide, we will investigate the different parts of way of life and sustenance that add to a better life. From taking on certain propensities to pursuing informed dietary decisions, these procedures can assist you with driving a more energetic and satisfying life.

Way of life Changes

Way of life changes are fundamental for working on by and large prosperity. These progressions envelop different parts of day to day existence, including active work, stress the executives, rest cleanliness, and social associations.

1. **Actual work:**

Actual work is a foundation of a sound way of life. Normal activity gives a large number of advantages, including worked on cardiovascular wellbeing, weight the board, and mental prosperity. Here are a few key contemplations:

1. **Sorts of Activity:** Consolidate a blend of high-impact (e.g., strolling, running, swimming) and strength-preparing works out (e.g., weightlifting, bodyweight works out) into your daily schedule.
2. **Consistency:** Hold back nothing 150 minutes of moderate-power oxygen consuming movement or 75 minutes of overwhelming force high-impact action each week, joined with muscle-fortifying exercises on at least two days per week.
3. **Assortment:** Stir up your exercises to forestall weariness and guarantee that different muscle bunches are locked in.
4. **Adaptability and Equilibrium:** Incorporate exercises like yoga or Pilates to further develop adaptability and equilibrium, lessening the gamble of injury.

2. Stress The executives:

1. **Care and Reflection:** Practice care to remain present and develop a quiet brain. Reflection methods can lessen pressure and tension.
2. **Breathing Activities:** Profound breathing activities, for example, diaphragmatic breathing or the 4-7-8 method, can rapidly quiet the sensory system.
3. **Using time productively:** Arrange your timetable to decrease the sensation of being overpowered. Focus on errands and agent when essential.
4. **Look for Help:** Make it a point to out to companions, family, or a psychological well-being proficient for help and direction.

3. Rest Cleanliness:

1. **Reliable Timetable:** Keep an ordinary rest plan by heading to sleep and awakening simultaneously consistently, even on ends of the week.

2. **Rest Climate:** Establish an agreeable and helpful rest climate, including a dim, calm, and cool room.

3. **Limit Screen Time:** Stay away from screens (telephones, PCs, televisions) before sleep time, as the blue light produced can upset the rest wake cycle.

4. **Limit Caffeine and Liquor:** Diminish caffeine and liquor admission, particularly at night, as they can disrupt rest.

4. Social Associations:

1. **Sustain Connections:** Put time and exertion in building and keeping up with positive associations with loved ones.

2. **Join Clubs or Gatherings:** Take part in exercises or clubs that line up with your inclinations to meet new individuals and encourage associations.

3. **Volunteer:** Chipping in benefits others as well as gives a feeling of motivation and local area.

Dietary Contemplations

Nourishment assumes an essential part in keeping up with well-being and forestalling persistent sicknesses. Settling on informed dietary decisions is fundamental for accomplishing ideal prosperity.

5. Adjusted Diet:

A decent eating routine furnishes the body with the essential supplements for development, fix, and support. Here are a few vital standards to keep:

1. **Assortment:** Eat a wide assortment of food sources, including organic products, vegetables, entire grains, lean proteins, and sound fats.

2. **Segment Control:** Be aware of piece sizes to forestall indulging and keep a solid weight.

3. **Limit Handled Food varieties:** Limit the utilization of handled food sources high in added sugars, salt, and undesirable fats.

4. **Remain Hydrated:** Drink a lot of water over the course of the day to help different physical processes.

6. Macronutrients:

1. **Starches:** Pick complex carbs like entire grains, natural products, and vegetables over refined sugars and white flour items.

2. **Proteins:** Incorporate lean protein sources like poultry, fish, beans, and tofu in your eating regimen to help muscle wellbeing and tissue fix.

3. **Fats:** Spotlight on solid fats like those tracked down in avocados, nuts, seeds, and olive oil while restricting soaked and trans fats.

7. Micronutrients:

1. **Nutrients:** Consume various beautiful leafy foods to get a range of nutrients, and consider nutrient enhancements whenever prompted by a medical care proficient.

2. **Minerals:** Consolidate mineral-rich food sources like dairy items, mixed greens, and nuts into your eating routine.

8. Exceptional Dietary Contemplations:

1. **Food Sensitivities and Prejudices:** Distinguish and keep away from food sources that trigger sensitivities or bigotries. Counsel a medical care proficient for direction.

2. **Veggie lover or Vegetarian Diets:** Plan adjusted eats less that give fundamental supplements, including vitamin B12, iron, and protein.

3. **Without gluten Diet:** Assuming you have celiac infection or gluten awareness, pick sans gluten grains like rice, quinoa, and oats.

9. Hydration:

1. **Day to day Admission:** Mean to drink somewhere around eight 8-ounce glasses of water each day (around 2 liters), and change in view of your action level and environment.
2. **Hydrating Food varieties:** Drink water-rich food sources like products of the soil to add to your day to day hydration.

10. Careful Eating:

1. **Eat Without Interruptions:** Try not to eat before the television or PC. Center around the taste, surface, and smell of your food.
2. **Pay attention to Craving Prompts:** Focus on your body's yearning and completion signs to forestall indulging.
3. **Bite Completely:** Bite your food gradually and completely to help processing and upgrade supplement ingestion.

Executing Way of life and Healthful Changes
Stage 1: Self-Evaluation:

1. Check out your ongoing way of life and dietary propensities.
2. Recognize regions where you might want to make enhancements.
3. Put forth sensible objectives that are explicit, quantifiable, and attainable.

Stage 2: Training:

1. Instruct yourself about good dieting and way of life decisions.

2. Counsel dependable sources, like enlisted dietitians and medical services experts.

Stage 3: Progressive Changes:

1. Begin by making little, sensible changes to your everyday practice.
2. For instance, increment your everyday vegetable admission or focus on a 10-minute day to day reflection practice.

Stage 4: Arranging:

1. Plan your dinners and snacks ahead of time to guarantee adjusted sustenance.
2. Make a week after week feast plan and staple rundown to stay away from rash food decisions.

Stage 5: Responsibility:

1. Share your objectives with a companion or relative who can offer help and consolation.
2. Think about keeping a diary to keep tabs on your development.

Stage 6: Look for Proficient Direction:

1. On the off chance that you have explicit dietary worries or medical issue, counsel an enrolled dietitian or medical care supplier for customized guidance.

6

Chapter 6

Improving Coordination

Coordination is the capacity to play out numerous assignments easily and effectively, including the synchronization of physical and mental cycles. Whether it's strolling, moving, playing an instrument, or succeeding in sports, coordination assumes a significant part in our day to day routines. Further developing coordination can upgrade our exhibition in different exercises, forestall wounds, and lift by and large certainty.

This far reaching guide investigates the complexities of coordination, diving into its physical and mental angles. We will look at the elements that impact coordination, the significance of coordination in different spaces, and a large number of techniques and activities intended to assist you with upgrading your coordination capacities. Whether you're a competitor planning to succeed in your game, a performer trying to work on your playing, or somebody just hoping to turn out to be more dexterous and elegant in day to day existence, these methods can be custom fitted to your necessities.

Figuring out Coordination

Before we dive into techniques for further developing coordination, it's fundamental to comprehend what coordination envelops and the elements that impact it.

1.1 Meaning of Coordination

Coordination, from a wide perspective, alludes to the capacity to amicably incorporate different body parts and mental cycles to perform undertakings easily and successfully. This incorporates activities like strolling, running, getting a ball, playing an instrument, and in any event, composing on a console. Coordination includes the mind, muscles, joints, and tactile frameworks cooperating consistently.

1.2 Elements Influencing Coordination

A few elements impact coordination:

1. **Neurological Elements:** The mind and sensory system assume a focal part in coordination. Any neurological condition or injury can affect coordination.

2. **Muscle Strength and Adaptability:** Feeble or tight muscles can thwart coordination by restricting the scope of movement and command over body parts.

3. **Tangible Information:** Vision, proprioception (familiarity with body position), and vestibular capability (balance and spatial direction) are basic for coordination.

4. **Practice and Ability Advancement:** Coordination improves with training and reiteration. Abilities become more programmed with time and experience.

5. **Fixation and Concentration:** Mental cycles, like consideration and focus, are fundamental for coordination.

Coordination in Various Spaces

Coordination is certainly not a one-size-fits-all idea; it shows contrastingly in different spaces of life and exercises. Understanding how coordination applies to these spaces can assist you with fitting your endeavors to work on in unambiguous regions.

2.1 Games and Athletic Execution

In sports, coordination is key. It includes the exact timing of developments, equilibrium, and deftness. Competitors frequently take part in specific coordination preparing to succeed in their picked sports.

1. **Dexterity:** Sports like tennis, baseball, and table tennis require exact dexterity to hit a moving objective precisely.
2. **Footwork and Equilibrium:** Sports like soccer, tumbling, and dance depend vigorously on facilitated footwork and equilibrium.
3. **Response Time:** Fast response times are essential in sports like boxing, hand to hand fighting, and b-ball.

2.2 Music and Performing Expressions

Artists, artists, and entertainers depend on coordination to make an agreeable and expressive presentation.

1. **Instrumental Coordination:** Artists should arrange their fingers, hands, and breath to create music.
2. **Dance Coordination:** Artists require exact coordination of developments, mood, and articulation.
3. **Acting and Feeling:** Entertainers need to facilitate actual motions, discourse, and feelings to convincingly depict characters.

2.3 Regular Exercises

In day to day existence, coordination is fundamental for errands going from driving a vehicle to composing on a console or in any event, preparing a feast.

1. **Fine Coordinated movements:** Exercises like composing, utilizing cutlery, and tying shoestrings include fine engine coordination.

2. **Gross Coordinated movements:** Strolling, climbing steps, and lifting objects require composed gross coordinated movements.

3. **Performing various tasks:** Planning different errands at the same time, for example, cooking while at the same time speaking, exhibits mental and actual coordination.

Techniques for Further developing Coordination

Now that we comprehend the meaning of coordination and its different applications, we should investigate techniques and activities to improve this essential expertise.

3.1 Actual Coordination Activities

1. **Balance Activities:** Equilibrium sheets, strength balls, and yoga presents like tree posture or champion posture can further develop equilibrium and proprioception.

2. **Strength Preparing:** Developing muscle fortitude through weightlifting or bodyweight practices improves by and large actual coordination.

3. **Practical Developments:** Consolidate useful developments like squats, lurches, and boards into your exercise routine daily schedule to further develop coordination in ordinary exercises.

4. **Deftness Drills:** Dexterity stepping stool drills, cone bores, and transport runs upgrade spryness and coordination in sports.

5. **Dance and Combative techniques:** Taking part in dance classes or hand to hand fighting disciplines, for example, capoeira or taekwondo, can fundamentally further develop coordination.

3.2 Mental Coordination Activities

1. **Mental Difficulties:** Participate in puzzles, entertaining riddles, and memory games to help mental coordination.

2. **Double Undertaking Preparing:** Work on performing two errands at the same time, like tackling numerical statements while strolling or talking.

3. **Response Time Drills:** Use response time applications and activities to work on your mental coordination.

4. **Visual Insight Preparing:** Improve visual coordination through exercises like following moving articles or perceiving designs.

3.3 Broadly educating

Broadly educating includes partaking in assorted exercises to work on generally coordination.

1. **Sports and Leisure activities:** Investigate different games and side interests to challenge various parts of coordination.

2. **Blended Exercises:** Consolidate exercises like swimming, yoga, and strength preparing to draw in both physical and mental coordination.

3. **Multidisciplinary Preparing:** Exploit multidisciplinary programs that consolidate physical and mental components, for example, parkour or deterrent course dashing.

3.4 Coordination Preparing Projects

Organized coordination preparing programs, frequently planned by wellness experts or mentors, can offer a precise way to deal with progress.

1. **Sport-Explicit Preparation:** Competitors frequently follow specific coordination preparing programs custom fitted to their games.

2. **Dance and Music Schooling:** Formal preparation in dance and music includes moderate coordination activities and schedules.

3. **Recovery Projects:** For people recuperating from wounds or neurological circumstances, restoration programs center around reestablishing coordination.

3.5 Care and Brain Body Practices

Care rehearses improve mind-body coordination by advancing mindfulness and concentration.

1. **Contemplation:** Care reflection further develops focus and mental coordination.
2. **Judo and Qigong:** These psyche body rehearses accentuate slow, purposeful developments that improve physical and mental coordination.

Integrating Coordination Preparing into Your Life

Further developing coordination is a continuous interaction that requires devotion and consistency. Here is a bit by bit way to deal with integrating coordination preparing into your day to day routine:

4.1 Survey Your Coordination Abilities

1. Recognize weak spots or explicit exercises where you might want to further develop coordination.
2. Think about looking for proficient direction or appraisal, particularly assuming you have explicit objectives or limits.

4.2 Put forth Clear Objectives

1. Characterize clear, reachable objectives for your coordination improvement venture.
2. Separate long haul objectives into more modest, sensible achievements.

4.3 Make a Customized Plan

1. Pick coordination activities and exercises that line up with your objectives and interests.
2. Foster an organized preparation plan that incorporates a blend of physical, mental, and broadly educating works out.

4.4 Timetable Normal Practice

1. Devote time to rehearse coordination practices routinely. Consistency is vital to progress.
2. Integrate coordination preparing into your everyday practice, whether it's during exercises, leisure activities, or day to day assignments.

4.5 Look for Proficient Direction

1. Think about working with a wellness mentor, mentor, or expert in your picked movement to plan a customized coordination preparing program.
2. In the event that you have explicit dexterity difficulties or constraints, talk with a medical services proficient or actual specialist.

4.6 Screen Progress and Adjust

1. Keep tabs on your development routinely to survey upgrades and make vital changes in accordance with your preparation plan.
2. Be patient and perceive that coordination improvement might require some investment, particularly for complex abilities.

6.1 Coordination-building exercises and drills.

Coordination is a basic expertise that impacts our capacity to perform different physical and mental undertakings easily and productively. Whether you're a competitor planning to succeed in your game, a performer hoping to work on your playing, or somebody who basically needs to upgrade your regular coordination, there are explicit activities and drills that can assist you with accomplishing your objectives.

This exhaustive aide centers around coordination-building activities and drills. We will investigate a great many exercises intended to upgrade both physical and mental coordination. These activities can be adjusted to suit people of any age and expertise levels, making them open to anybody looking to further develop their coordination capacities.

Actual Coordination Activities

Actual coordination includes the synchronization of developments and body parts to productively perform undertakings. Here are a few activities and drills to assist you with building actual coordination:

1.1 Equilibrium Activities:

Balance is an essential part of coordination, particularly in sports and exercises that require soundness and control. These activities advance equilibrium and proprioception (familiarity with body position).

Practice 1.1.1 - Single-Leg Equilibrium:

Stand on one leg with your other foot somewhat off the ground.

Keep your arms at your sides or put your hands on your hips.

Attempt to keep up with your equilibrium for 30 seconds to a moment.

Change to the next leg and rehash.

Practice 1.1.2 - Yoga Tree Posture:

Stand on one leg with your other foot put against your inward thigh.

Unite your hands before your chest in a request position.

Center around a guide before you toward assist with balance.

Hold the posture for 30 seconds to a moment.

Change to the next leg.

1.2 Dexterity Activities:

Dexterity is vital in exercises like games, playing instruments, and, surprisingly, regular assignments like composing. These activities work on the association between your visual discernment and hand developments.

Practice 1.2.1 - Shuffling:

Begin with two balls or objects of equivalent weight.

Throw one ball from one hand to the next in a bend.

As it drops, throw the second ball from the other hand to make a nonstop beat.

Slowly add more balls as you become more capable.

Practice 1.2.2 - Tennis Ball Bobbing:

Stand confronting a wall with a tennis ball in one hand.

Toss the ball against the wall, permitting it to quickly return.

Get the ball with a similar hand you tossed it with.

Rehash this interaction, going for the gold and reliable mood.

1.3 Dexterity and Footwork Drills:

Many games and proactive tasks require fast shifts in course and exact footwork. These drills work on your capacity to move rapidly and effectively.

Practice 1.3.1 - Cone Drills:

Set up a progression of cones in an orderly fashion with around 1-2 feet between them.

Start toward one side and wind through the cones as fast as could be expected, crisscrossing from one side to another.

As you arrive at the end, invert bearing and wind back through the cones.

Practice 1.3.2 - Parallel Mix:

Stand with your feet shoulder-width separated.

Mix sideways to one side for a couple of steps, keeping your knees marginally twisted.

Then, at that point, mix to one side for similar number of steps.

Rehash this sidelong mix for 30 seconds to a moment.

Mental Coordination Activities

Mental coordination includes the synchronization of mental capabilities like consideration, memory, and critical thinking with actual activities. Here are activities to work on mental coordination:

2.1 Memory and Development Coordination:

These activities challenge your memory and capacity to facilitate developments in light of guidelines or groupings.

Practice 2.1.1 - Simon Says:

Pick one individual to be the pioneer (Simon).

The pioneer provides orders like "Simon says contact your toes" or "Simon expresses bounce on one foot."

Members should possibly follow the order assuming that it starts with "Simon says."

In the event that the pioneer provides an order without saying "Simon says" first, anybody who follows is out.

Go on until just a single individual remaining parts.

Practice 2.1.2 - Memory Succession Game:

Make a grouping of developments or activities, like applauding, stepping, or contacting different body parts.

Begin with a basic succession and increment the intricacy as you progress.

One individual plays out the grouping, and the following individual rehashes it and adds another activity.

Go on until somebody neglects or commits an error.

2.2 Response Time and Coordination:

Further developing response time is fundamental in exercises like games and driving. These activities upgrade your capacity to respond rapidly and precisely.

Practice 2.2.1 - Ball Drop Test:

Stand confronting an accomplice who holds a tennis ball or little item at shoulder level.

The accomplice fails all of a sudden, and you should get it as fast as could be expected.

Rehash with varieties like utilizing different hand positions or getting with one hand.

Practice 2.2.2 - Response Time Application:

Download a response time application on your cell phone or tablet.

These applications regularly include tapping the screen in light of a visual or hear-able sign as fast as could really be expected.

Challenge yourself to further develop your response time after some time.

2.3 Double Assignment Preparing:

Double errand preparing includes performing at least two assignments all the while, testing your mental and actual coordination.

Practice 2.3.1 - Strolling and then some:

Stroll in an orderly fashion while counting in reverse from 100 by deducting 7 (e.g., 100, 93, 86, and so forth.).

This exercise tests your capacity to keep up with balance and mental concentration while strolling.

Practice 2.3.2 - Shuffling and then some:

While shuffling balls or beanbags, count without holding back or present a sonnet.

Shuffling requires dexterity, and counting adds a mental test.

Consolidating Physical and Mental Coordination

Numerous exercises require the incorporation of physical and mental coordination. Here are practices that join the two perspectives:

3.1 Kendo:

Kendo is a brain body practice that underlines slow, streaming developments, controlled breathing, and care. It improves actual co-ordination while advancing mental concentration and unwinding.

Practice 3.1.1 - Jujitsu Essential Developments:

Learn and rehearse essential Judo developments, for example, "Cloud Hands" or "Brush Knee and Bend Step."

Center around the smoothness of your developments, planning them with profound, cadenced relaxing.

3.2 Dance:

Moving includes exact body developments, cadence, and coordination with music. It's an amazing method for improving both physical and mental coordination.

Practice 3.2.1 - Dance Schedule:

Pick a dance style that intrigues you, whether it's dance hall, hip-jump, salsa, or artful dance.

Become familiar with a dance routine or movement, focusing on the synchronization of developments with music.

3.3 Games Explicit Drills:

For competitors, sports-explicit drills work on actual coordination as well as improve mental abilities connected with the game.

Practice 3.3.1 - Ball Passing Drill:

Set up a passing drill where you pass the b-ball to an accomplice while moving around the court.

Integrate spilling and shooting into the drill to mimic genuine game situations.

Practice 3.3.2 - Soccer Spilling and Independent direction:

Work on spilling a soccer ball through cones while coming to fast conclusions about when to pass or head in a different path.

This drill improves both ball control and mental navigation.

Integrating Coordination Preparing into Day to day existence

Further developing coordination is a continuous cycle that requires reliable practice and combination into your day to day daily schedule. This is the way to integrate coordination preparing into your life:

4.1 Put forth Unambiguous Objectives:

1. Recognize areas of coordination you need to improve, whether it's equilibrium, dexterity, or response time.
2. Put forth clear and quantifiable objectives to keep tabs on your development.

4.2 Make an Organized Arrangement:

1. Foster a preparation plan that incorporates a blend of activities and drills custom fitted to your objectives.
2. Plan explicit times for coordination preparing inside your week by week schedule.

4.3 Beginning with a Warm-up:

1. Start every coordination meeting with an intensive get ready to set up your body and brain for the activities.
2. Incorporate dynamic stretches and light high-impact exercises to increment blood stream.

4.4 Consistency is Critical:

1. Commit normal opportunity to coordination preparing, going for the gold a couple of meetings each week.
2. Bit by bit increment the intricacy and power of activities as you progress.

4.5 Look for Proficient Direction:

1. Think about working with a mentor, coach, or educator who has practical experience in practical dexterity preparing, particularly on the off chance that you have explicit objectives or constraints.
2. They can give significant criticism and modify your preparation program.

4.6 Screen Progress:

1. Keep a preparation diary to record your activities, upgrades, and difficulties.
2. Routinely survey your diary to evaluate your advancement and change your arrangement likewise.

4.7 Stay Careful:

1. Focus on your body and brain during coordination works out.

2. Care improves your attention to developments and refines your coordination.

6.2 Integrating coordination into daily activities.

Coordination is a central expertise that impacts our capacity to perform different undertakings proficiently and successfully. While many individuals partner coordination fundamentally with sports or melodic exercises, it assumes a huge part in regular day to day existence. The manner in which we move, connect with our current circumstance, and even cycle data includes coordination. In this manner, coordinating coordination into everyday exercises can prompt better actual wellness, mental capability, and by and large prosperity.

In this complete aide, we will investigate the idea of incorporating coordination into day to day existence. We will dive into the significance of coordination in different parts of regular exercises and give reasonable techniques to improve physical and mental abilities. Whether you are a competitor hoping to upgrade your presentation, an understudy looking for further developed concentration and efficiency, or essentially somebody keen on living a more planned and satisfying life, this guide is for you.

The Significance of Coordination in Day to day existence

Coordination is something beyond the capacity to perform complex actual developments; it stretches out to mental capabilities, performing various tasks, and

flexibility. Understanding the meaning of coordination in ordinary exercises is the most vital move toward integrating it into your everyday daily practice.

1.1 Actual Coordination in Day to day existence:

1. **Versatility and Equilibrium:** Strolling, climbing steps, and exploring hindrances require coordination between appendages, muscles, and the tangible framework.

2. **Fine Coordinated movements:** Assignments like composition, composing, and utilizing utensils depend on exact dexterity and mastery.

3. **Wellbeing and Anticipation:** Coordination is fundamental for keeping away from mishaps, for example, stumbling and falling or spilling hot fluids.

1.2 Mental Coordination in Day to day existence:

Mental coordination includes the synchronization of mental cycles, for example,

1. **Consideration and Concentration:** Keeping up with focus on undertakings, whether perusing, examining, or working, is a type of mental coordination.

2. **Performing multiple tasks:** Proficiently dealing with different errands and exchanging between them requires mental coordination.

3. **Critical thinking:** Organizing mental cycles to break down and take care of issues is a principal part of regular day to day existence.

1.3 Profound Coordination in Day to day existence:

1. **Close to home Guideline:** Planning feelings to answer suitably to various circumstances is pivotal for keeping up with sound connections and mental prosperity.

2. **Sympathy and Correspondence:** Powerful correspondence depends on grasping others' feelings and conveying one's own considerations and sentiments intelligibly.

Techniques for Incorporating Coordination into Day to day Exercises

Now that we perceive the significance of coordination in day to day existence, we should investigate systems for consistently integrating coordination-incorporating exercises into your everyday practice.

2.1 Actual Coordination in Day to day Exercises:

Upgrading actual coordination in day to day existence can prompt superior versatility, equilibrium, and generally wellness. Here are pragmatic procedures to accomplish this:

Methodology 2.1.1 - Dynamic Driving:

Pick dynamic methods of driving, like strolling or cycling, whenever the situation allows.

These exercises connect with your lower body muscles and further develop equilibrium and coordination.

Technique 2.1.2 - Family Tasks:

View family tasks as any open doors for actual coordination works out.

Undertakings like vacuuming, clearing, and cultivating include a scope of developments that upgrade coordination.

Methodology 2.1.3 - Wellness Breaks:

Integrate short wellness breaks into your typical business day.

Perform fast coordination works out, for example, balance difficulties or bodyweight developments, to separate delayed times of sitting.

2.2 Mental Coordination in Day to day Exercises:

Procedure 2.2.1 - Using time productively:

Use time usage methods, like the Pomodoro Procedure, to structure your business day.

This strategy includes rotating centered work spans with brief breaks, advancing mental coordination and efficiency.

System 2.2.2 - Careful Exercises:

Participate in care rehearses like contemplation or profound breathing activities.

These exercises upgrade mental coordination via preparing your brain to remain present and centered.

System 2.2.3 - Puzzles:

Commit a couple of moments every day to tackle riddles, puzzles, or challenging yet fun riddles.

These difficulties animate mental coordination and critical thinking abilities.

2.3 Profound Coordination in Day to day Exercises:

Successful close to home coordination can prompt better connections and in general profound prosperity. This is the way to accomplish it:

Procedure 2.3.1 - Undivided attention:

Practice undivided attention while taking part in discussions.

Give close consideration to others' feelings, nonverbal signals, and words to compassionately answer.

System 2.3.2 - Compromise:

Foster compromise abilities to usefully deal with conflicts.

This includes organizing feelings, correspondence, and critical thinking to arrive at commonly useful arrangements.

Everyday Exercises for Upgrading Coordination

3.1 Strolling and Running:

1. **Strolling:** Spotlight on keeping a lively speed, swinging your arms normally, and focusing on your stance.
2. **Running:** Step by step increment the intricacy by integrating time periods, running, or in any event, running on lopsided landscape for improved balance.

3.2 Preparing and Feast Arrangement:

1. **Cleaving Vegetables:** Utilize a blade capably to dice, hack, and julienne vegetables, upgrading dexterity.
2. **Timing:** Coordinate cooking times for different parts of a feast, like pasta, sauce, and vegetables.

3. **Performing various tasks:** At the same time set up numerous dishes or handle different cooking strategies, testing mental coordination.

3.3 Playing Instruments:

1. **Console Instruments:** Playing the piano or console includes planning hand developments, finger finesse, and perusing printed music.
2. **String Instruments:** Instruments like the guitar or violin request exact coordination between finger position, playing, and music translation.
3. **Wind Instruments:** Playing wind instruments requires synchronizing finger developments, breath control, and note perusing.

3.4 Planting:

1. **Digging and Planting:** Use cultivating instruments with accuracy, sowing seeds or bulbs at the right profundity and distance.
2. **Arranging and Association:** Coordinate the design of your nursery, choosing viable plants and arranging occasional consideration schedules.
3. **Profound Coordination:** Sustain your plants by giving satisfactory consideration, answering their requirements, and encountering the delight of development.

3.5 Yoga and Kendo:

1. **Yoga:** Participate in yoga represents that challenge equilibrium, adaptability, and focus, for example, tree posture or champion posture.
2. **Jujitsu:** Practice slow, streaming developments that blend physical and mental coordination, advancing unwinding and care.

Day to day Daily schedule for Upgraded Coordination
4.1 Morning Schedule:

1. **Equilibrium and Versatility Activities:** Begin your day with straightforward equilibrium practices like remaining on one leg or performing lower leg circles.
2. **Careful Relaxing:** Practice profound breathing activities to improve center and mental coordination.
3. **Fine Coordinated movements:** Participate in exercises like stringing a needle or settling a little riddle to further develop dexterity.

4.2 Work or School Day:

1. **Dynamic Driving:** If conceivable, walk or bicycle to work or school to take part in actual coordination exercises.
2. **Booked Breaks:** Integrate short coordination activities or entertaining puzzles during breaks to support mental coordination.
3. **Careful Eating:** Focus on your dietary patterns, relishing each nibble, and rehearsing close to home coordination with your food decisions.

4.3 Night Schedule:

1. **Preparing Supper:** Use dinner arrangement as a chance to upgrade coordination through slashing, performing multiple tasks, and timing.
2. **Music or Craftsmanship:** Invest some energy playing an instrument, drawing, or participating in imaginative exercises to work on fine coordinated movements.
3. **Reflect and Loosen up:** Think about your day, recognizing your close to home coordination endeavors in different associations.

4.4 Sleep time Schedule:

1. **Extending and Unwinding:** Perform delicate stretches or partake in unwinding works out, like Kendo or reflection, to loosen up and advance mental coordination.
2. **Journaling:** Write in a diary to consider your day to day coordination accomplishments, regions for development, and objectives for the following day.

Chapter 7

Lifespan Considerations

Life is a wonderful excursion that unfurls from the snapshot of birth and go on through different stages until the inescapable course of maturing. Each period of life brings its interesting difficulties, delights, and achievements. Life expectancy contemplations envelop the physical, mental, close to home, and social viewpoints that advance as people progress through earliest stages, youth, immaturity, adulthood, and into their later years.

This far reaching guide investigates life expectancy contemplations, revealing insight into the various phases of human turn of events and the different variables that impact our prosperity at each stage. We will dive into the basic components that influence actual wellbeing, mental prosperity, and generally speaking personal satisfaction all through the life expectancy. By understanding these contemplations, people can pursue informed choices and explore the excursion of existence with more prominent strength and satisfaction.

Earliest stages and Youth

The underlying long periods of life are set apart by quick development and improvement. During earliest stages and youth, people experience amazing physical and mental changes, establishing the groundwork for their future.

1.1 Actual Turn of events:

1. **Coordinated abilities:** Babies progressively foster their gross and fine coordinated movements, advancing from straightforward developments like turning over to slithering, strolling, and in the end running.
2. **Development:** Fast actual development is obvious as babies put on weight and length during their initial not many years.
3. **Tactile Turn of events:** Tangible frameworks, including vision, hearing, and contact, mature, permitting babies to investigate their current circumstance.

1.2 Mental Turn of events:

1. **Mental Achievements:** Kids create essential mental abilities like item changelessness (understanding that articles exist in any event, when concealed) and representative play.
2. **Language Procurement:** Language abilities progress, with youngsters commonly arriving at huge language achievements, such as framing sentences, during this period.
3. **Social and Close to home Turn of events:** Newborn children and babies structure connections to parental figures, experience feelings, and start to foster compassion.

1.3 Social and Close to home Turn of events:

1. **Connection:** The development of secure connections with guardians is significant for close to home prosperity.
2. **Feeling Guideline:** Kids figure out how to perceive and deal with their feelings, with help from guardians.

3. **Play and Socialization:** Play assists kids with creating interactive abilities and investigate their inventiveness.

Youth and Pre-adulthood

As youngsters progress into youth and immaturity, they keep on encountering critical development, both actually and intellectually. These stages bring new difficulties, instructive open doors, and social elements.

2.1 Actual Turn of events:

1. **Pubescence:** Immaturity is set apart by the beginning of adolescence, acquiring changes auxiliary sexual attributes and fast development.
2. **Actual Wellness:** Commitment to proactive tasks becomes significant for developing fortitude, perseverance, and coordination.
3. **Nourishment:** Youths require adjusted sustenance to help their development and improvement.

2.2 Mental Turn of events:

1. **Unique Reasoning:** Teenagers begin thinking all the more dynamically and foster decisive reasoning abilities.
2. **Scholarly Accomplishment:** Instructive open doors become focal, with understudies confronting expanding scholastic requests.
3. **Character Development:** Youths investigate their personality, values, and convictions.

2.3 Social and Profound Turn of events:

1. **Peer Connections:** Companionships and friend collaborations assume a critical part in friendly turn of events.
2. **Close to home Guideline:** Youths refine their profound guideline abilities.

3. **Independence and Freedom:** As kids develop, they look for more prominent independence and autonomy from their guardians.

Adulthood

Adulthood is a different stage described by different life altering situations, obligations, and self-improvement. It tends to be additionally partitioned into right on time, center, and late adulthood.

3.1 Early Adulthood:

1. **Training and Vocation:** People seek after advanced education, lay out professions, and go with significant decisions.
2. **Close connections:** Arrangement of close connections and choices in regards to marriage and family happen.
3. **Actual Wellbeing:** Keeping up with actual wellness and prosperity turns out to be progressively significant.

3.2 Center Adulthood:

1. **Vocation Advancement:** Numerous people arrive at the pinnacle of their professions during this stage.
2. **Everyday Life:** Bringing up kids, sustaining connections, and potentially encountering the "unfilled home" condition.
3. **Actual Changes:** Maturing related actual changes become more observable, requiring consideration regarding wellbeing and health.

3.3 Late Adulthood:

1. **Retirement:** Numerous people resign from their vocations and enter another period of life.
2. **Wellbeing Difficulties:** Maturing frequently brings wellbeing challenges, requiring clinical consideration and way of life changes.

3. **Mental Changes:** A few mental changes might happen, yet numerous more seasoned grown-ups keep up with smartness and learn.

Improving with age

Maturing is a characteristic piece of life, and improving with age includes embracing the interaction while keeping up with physical and mental prosperity.

4.1 Actual Wellbeing:

1. **Work out:** Ordinary active work, including strength preparing and cardiovascular activity, keeps up with bulk, adaptability, and by and large wellbeing.
2. **Nourishment:** A fair eating regimen wealthy in natural products, vegetables, lean proteins, and entire grains upholds actual wellbeing and decreases the gamble of constant sicknesses.
3. **Preventive Consideration:** Customary check-ups and screenings can get medical problems early, expanding the possibilities of effective therapy.

4.2 Mental Prosperity:

1. **Mental Commitment:** Kept learning, mental excitement, and exercises like riddles or games assist with keeping up with mental capability.
2. **Social Associations:** Keeping up with social connections and taking part in local area exercises battle depression and advance close to home prosperity.
3. **Close to home Wellbeing:** Practices like care, reflection, and directing can assist with overseeing pressure and keep up with profound wellbeing.

4.3 Monetary Preparation:

1. **Retirement Arranging:** Cautious monetary preparation, including reserve funds and ventures, guarantees monetary security in retirement.
2. **Domain Arranging:** Making a will and making game plans for the dispersion of resources and medical services choices is fundamental.

4.4 Personal satisfaction:

1. **Seek after Interests:** Participating in leisure activities, interests, and exercises that give pleasure and satisfaction improves life.
2. **Remain Inquisitive:** An inquisitive and open outlook cultivates long lasting learning and self-awareness.
3. **Encouraging groups of people:** Rest on encouraging groups of people, including loved ones, to explore the difficulties of maturing.

Life expectancy Contemplations in Contemporary Society
5.1 Innovative Headways:

1. **Medical services:** Advances in medical services innovation offer better finding and therapy choices, expanding life expectancy and working on personal satisfaction.
2. **Correspondence:** Innovation interfaces individuals across ages, taking into consideration more prominent communication and backing.

5.2 Training and Vocation:

1. **Deep rooted Learning:** Long lasting learning valuable open doors are more available than any other time, permitting people to proceed with their schooling and expertise improvement.

5.3 Social Elements:

1. **Multigenerational Families:** Numerous families are made out of different ages, encouraging intergenerational connections and backing.

7.1 Addressing balance and coordination in different life stages.
Equilibrium and coordination are basic parts of human development and usefulness. All through our lives, from outset to advanced age, the capacity to keep up with equilibrium and direction our developments assumes a basic part in day to day exercises, actual wellness, and generally prosperity. This extensive aide will investigate how equilibrium and coordination advance across various life stages, from outset to late adulthood. We will examine the special difficulties and contemplations at each stage and give useful systems to upgrade and address these viewpoints over the course of life.

Outset and Youth
The excursion of creating equilibrium and coordination starts in outset and youth. This stage is set apart by quick physical and mental development, establishing the groundwork for future development and coordinated abilities.

1.1 Actual Turn of events:

1. **Engine Achievements:** Babies progress from straightforward reflexive developments to turning over, slithering, and in the end strolling.
2. **Tactile Coordination:** The faculties, like vision, hearing, and proprioception, assume a critical part in early actual turn of events.

1.2 Mental and Engine Coordination:

1. **Coming to and Getting a handle on:** Babies figure out how to go after items and direction their hand developments to get a handle on them.
2. **Exploratory Developments:** Early developments are exploratory, assisting newborn children with finding out about their current circumstance and foster coordination.
3. **Tactile Input:** Tangible criticism assists babies with refining their coordinated abilities and figure out how to control their developments.

1.3 Difficulties and Methodologies:

1. **Oversight:** Newborn children require steady management to guarantee their wellbeing as they investigate their environmental factors.
2. **Belly Time:** Urge stomach time to advance the improvement of neck and chest area
strength, which is fundamental for creeping and later strolling.
3. **Play and Development:** Give chances to play that include coming to, snatching, and investigating objects to encourage coordination.

Youth and Puberty

During youth and puberty, the improvement of equilibrium and coordination turns out to be more refined as kids take part in different proactive tasks and sports.

2.1 Actual Turn of events:

1. **Development Sprays:** Youths might encounter development sprays that briefly influence their coordination and equilibrium.
2. **Pubescence:** Hormonal changes can impact actual turn of events, including muscle development and body sythesis.

2.2 Coordinated abilities and Sports:

1. **Sports Cooperation:** Kids and teenagers frequently partake in coordinated sports, which require explicit equilibrium and coordination abilities.
2. **Engine Expertise Refinement:** Exercises like riding a bicycle, swimming, and playing group activities advance coordination and equilibrium.

2.3 Difficulties and Systems:

1. **Injury Anticipation:** Young people are in danger of sports-related wounds because of their support in proactive tasks. Appropriate warm-up, molding, and method are fundamental.
2. **Expertise Improvement:** Empower support in various exercises to foster many coordinated abilities and coordination capacities.
3. **Actual work:** Guarantee that kids and teenagers participate in standard active work to help the improvement of equilibrium and coordination.

Adulthood

In adulthood, keeping up with equilibrium and coordination becomes crucial for day to day exercises, actual wellness, and injury anticipation.

3.1 Actual Turn of events:

1. **Muscle Strength:** Keeping up with muscle strength is critical for equilibrium and coordination as people age.
2. **Joint Wellbeing:** Appropriate joint capability is fundamental for equilibrium and coordination.

3.2 Work and Way of life:

1. **Word related Requests:** A few occupations might require explicit coordination abilities, like those in development, medical care, or the performing expressions.
2. **Inactive Way of life:** Delayed sitting and a stationary way of life can prompt muscle irregular characteristics and diminished coordination.

3.3 Difficulties and Methodologies:

1. **Work-out Everyday practice:** Take part in standard work-out schedules that incorporate strength preparing, balance activities, and adaptability work to keep up with actual coordination.
2. **Ergonomics:** Keep up with appropriate ergonomics at work and home to forestall muscle awkward nature and strain.
3. **Sound Way of life:** Embrace a solid way of life that incorporates adjusted sustenance, standard active work, and sufficient rest to help in general prosperity.

Late Adulthood

In late adulthood, equilibrium and coordination can be trying because of the normal maturing process, however proactive measures can assist with keeping up with these capacities.

4.1 Actual Turn of events:

1. **Maturing Impacts:** Maturing prompts changes in bulk, bone thickness, and joint adaptability, influencing equilibrium and coordination.
2. **Tactile Changes:** Changes in vision, hearing, and proprioception can affect coordination.

4.2 Everyday Exercises:

1. **Utilitarian Portability:** Keeping up with equilibrium and coordination is urgent for exercises of everyday living, like strolling, dressing, and cooking.
2. **Fall Chance:** Equilibrium issues increment the gamble of falls in more seasoned grown-ups, prompting likely wounds.

4.3 Difficulties and Techniques:

1. **Practice for Seniors:** Empower support in senior work out schedules that emphasis on equilibrium and coordination works out.
2. **Customary Wellbeing Exams:** Ordinary tests with medical services suppliers can help recognize and address balance-related issues.
3. **Home Wellbeing:** Change the home climate to lessen fall dangers, like introducing handrails and eliminating stumbling risks.
4. **Social Commitment:** Urge social exercises to keep up with mental and profound prosperity, which can in a roundabout way support actual coordination.

Long lasting Techniques for Equilibrium and Coordination
Notwithstanding age, people can carry out deep rooted techniques to help and upgrade their equilibrium and coordination.
5.1 Activity and Actual work:

1. **Strength Preparing:** Integrate strength preparing practices into your daily schedule to assemble and keep up with bulk.
2. **Balance Activities:** Practice balance works out, like remaining on one leg or yoga, to further develop equilibrium and dependability.
3. **Coordination Exercises:** Take part in exercises that challenge coordination, like moving or playing sports.

5.2 Sustenance and Hydration:

1. **Adjusted Diet:** Consume a reasonable eating routine wealthy in supplements to help muscle and joint wellbeing.
2. **Hydration:** Remain sufficiently hydrated to keep up with muscle and joint capability.

5.3 Ordinary Wellbeing Exams:

1. **Yearly Physicals:** Timetable customary exams with medical care suppliers to screen and address any equilibrium or coordination-related concerns.

5.4 Psyche Body Practices:

1. **Care:** Practice care procedures to further develop center and mental lucidity, by implication improving coordination.
2. **Yoga and Judo:** Take part as a main priority body rehearses like yoga and Kendo, which advance actual equilibrium and mental coordination.

7.2 Strategies for seniors to prevent falls and injuries.

As we age, the gamble of falls and wounds turns into a critical worry for seniors. Falls can prompt serious results, including cracks, head wounds, and a deficiency of freedom. In any case, many falls are preventable with the right techniques and safety measures set up. This exhaustive aide means to furnish seniors and their guardians

with fundamental data on fall anticipation. We will investigate the normal gamble factors for falls among seniors and give pragmatic procedures and activities to keep up with strength, equilibrium, and generally speaking prosperity.

Understanding the Gamble Variables

Prior to plunging into techniques for fall counteraction, it's critical to comprehend the gamble factors that make seniors more defenseless to falls.

1.1 Age-Related Changes:

1. **Muscle Shortcoming:** As we age, there is a characteristic decrease in bulk and strength, influencing steadiness and equilibrium.
2. **Equilibrium and Walk Changes:** Changes in stride and adjust can happen because old enough related muscle and joint changes.
3. **Vision Changes:** Age-related vision changes, like decreased profundity discernment and fringe vision, can add to falls.

1.2 Constant Ailments:

1. **Joint pain:** Agony and joint firmness related with joint inflammation can influence versatility and equilibrium.
2. **Neurological Circumstances:** Conditions like Parkinson's sickness can affect coordination and step.
3. **Meds:** Certain drugs, for example, narcotics and circulatory strain meds, can cause

discombobulation and influence balance.

1.3 Ecological Perils:

1. **Mess and Stumbling Dangers:** Lopsided deck, mess, and free floor coverings can expand the gamble of falls.
2. **Unfortunate Lighting:** Deficient lighting can make it hard to recognize deterrents and dangers.
3. **Absence of Assistive Gadgets:** The shortfall of handrails, snatch bars, and other assistive gadgets can present dangers.

Methodologies for Fall Avoidance

Now that we've distinguished the gamble factors, we should investigate procedures to forestall falls and wounds among seniors.

2.1 Home Security:

1. **Clean up:** Eliminate mess and hindrances from walkways to guarantee make ways.
2. **Secure Mats:** Secure free floor coverings with twofold sided tape or eliminate them through and through.
3. **Lighting:** Further develop lighting all through the home, especially in corridors, flights of stairs, and washrooms.
4. **Get Bars:** Introduce get bars in the restroom and close to steps for added help.
5. **Handrails:** Guarantee that handrails are safely secured along flights of stairs and open air pathways.

2.2 Normal Activity:

1. **Strength Preparing:** Participate in strength-preparing activities to further develop bulk and in general strength.
2. **Balance Activities:** Practice balance-improving activities like remaining on one leg or strolling heel to toe.
3. **Adaptability:** Integrate extending schedules to keep up with joint adaptability and scope of movement.

2.3 Medicine The executives:

1. **Prescription Survey:** Routinely audit meds with medical services suppliers to evaluate expected aftereffects and communications.
2. **Get some information about Other options:** Examine medicine choices with your medical care supplier assuming that you experience wooziness or equilibrium issues.

2.4 Vision Care:

1. **Standard Eye Tests:** Timetable ordinary eye tests to address vision changes and update remedies.
2. **Utilize Remedial Focal points:** Guarantee you wear endorsed eyeglasses or contact focal points reliably.
3. **Great Lighting:** Utilize fitting lighting, incorporating bifocals with worked in lighting for better perceivability.

2.5 Footwear:

1. **Appropriate Footwear:** Pick strong, well-fitting footwear with non-slip bottoms.
2. **Keep away from High Heels:** Try not to wear high heels or shoes with unfortunate curve support, which can influence soundness.

2.6 Assistive Gadgets:

1. **Strolling Helps:** If necessary, use strolling helps, for example, sticks or walkers to give soundness and backing.
2. **Fall Cautions:** Consider utilizing fall discovery gadgets or crisis ready frameworks.

2.7 Stay Hydrated:

1. **Legitimate Hydration:** Drink satisfactory liquids over the course of the day to forestall dazedness or unsteadiness.

2.8 Medicine The executives:

1. **Medicine Survey:** Consistently audit prescriptions with medical services suppliers to evaluate expected secondary effects and collaborations.

2. **Get some information about Other options:** Examine medicine choices with your medical services supplier assuming you experience unsteadiness or equilibrium issues.

Activities for Fall Anticipation
3.1 Leg Strength Activities:

1. **Leg Raises:** Clutch a solid surface for help and lift one leg aside, front, and back. Perform 10-15 reiterations on every leg.
2. **Squats:** Stand with feet shoulder-width separated and gradually bring down your body as though you're sitting once more into a seat. Keep your knees over your lower legs. Perform 10-15 reiterations.

3.2 Equilibrium Activities:

1. **One-Leg Stand:** Stand on one leg while clutching a steady surface. Attempt to adjust for 30 seconds on every leg.
2. **Impact point to-Toe Walk:** Stroll in an orderly fashion, setting the impact point of one foot straightforwardly before the toes of the other. Rehash for 10-15 stages.

3.3 Adaptability Activities:

1. **Neck Rolls:** Gradually slant your head forward, to the right, in reverse, and to the left, finishing a round trip. Rehash the other way.
2. **Shoulder Rolls:** Shrug your shoulders up toward your ears, then, at that point, roll them back and down. Rehash 10-15 times.

3.4 Center Reinforcing Activities:

1. **Boards:** Begin in a push-up position, yet with your weight on your lower arms and toes. Hold for 15-30 seconds, steadily expanding the term.
2. **Leg Raises:** Lie on your back with your arms at your sides. Lift your legs off the ground a couple inches, then, at that point, lower them. Perform 10-15 reiterations.

3.5 Kendo and Yoga:

1. **Kendo:** Judo is a low-influence, sluggish activity that advances equilibrium and coordination. Consider signing up for Kendo classes.
2. **Yoga:** Yoga offers a scope of equilibrium improving postures and stretches. Go to yoga classes intended for seniors or follow online instructional exercises.

Looking for Proficient Direction
4.1 Active recuperation:

1. **Actual Specialists:** Consider working with an actual advisor who can plan a customized practice program custom-made to your necessities.
2. **Fall Hazard Appraisal:** Actual specialists can perform fall risk evaluations and give proposals.

4.2 Drug Survey:

1. **Drug specialist Conference:** Timetable an interview with a drug specialist to survey your prescriptions for potential fall-related secondary effects or cooperations.
2. **Drug Changes:** Talk about the chance of medicine changes or options with your medical care supplier.

4.3 Vision and Hearing Checks:

1. **Customary Tests:** Timetable ordinary eye and hearing tests to address age-related changes in vision and hearing.

The Significance of Correspondence
5.1 Self-Evaluation:

1. **Self-Observing:** Know about any progressions in your equilibrium, strength, or coordination, and discuss these progressions with your medical care supplier.
2. **Fall History:** Illuminate your medical care supplier about any past falls or close falls.

5.2 Guardian Correspondence:

1. **Family and Guardians:** Impart your interests and fall counteraction procedures with relatives and parental figures to guarantee a protected climate.

Chapter 8

Achieving Balance in Life

In the present quick moving world, accomplishing balance in life has turned into a central objective for some people. Balance, in this specific situation, alludes to the agreeable mix of different parts of life, including work, family, connections, wellbeing, self-improvement, and recreation. It is the craft of shuffling numerous obligations and pursuits while keeping up with physical, profound, and mental prosperity. This complete aide investigates the significance of equilibrium throughout everyday life, the difficulties individuals face in accomplishing it, and viable systems to lead a more amicable and satisfying life.

The Meaning of Equilibrium Throughout everyday life

1.1 Actual Prosperity:

1. **Wellbeing and Life span:** Equilibrium advances actual wellbeing and life span by lessening pressure and forestalling burnout.
2. **Energy Levels:** Keeping up with balance guarantees higher energy levels, empowering you to really handle everyday difficulties.

1.2 Close to home Wellbeing:

1. **Stress Decrease:** Equilibrium diminishes feelings of anxiety, prompting better profound wellbeing and flexibility.
2. **Further developed Connections:** Close to home equilibrium cultivates better and additional satisfying associations with others.

1.3 Mental Lucidity:

1. **Upgraded Concentration:** Equilibrium considers better fixation and spotlight on undertakings, bringing about superior efficiency.
2. **Imagination and Critical thinking:** A reasonable psyche is more innovative and powerful in critical thinking.

\

1.4 Satisfaction and Fulfillment:

1. **Feeling of Direction:** Equilibrium assists people adjust their activities to their qualities, prompting a more prominent feeling of direction and satisfaction.
2. **Balanced Life:** A healthy lifestyle offers potential open doors for self-improvement, investigation, and self-revelation.

Normal Difficulties to Accomplishing Equilibrium
2.1 Work-Life Unevenness:

1. **Long Working Hours:** Many individuals face requesting work plans that allow for different parts of life.
2. **Business related Pressure:** Elevated degrees of business related pressure can gush out over into individual life, influencing generally speaking equilibrium.

2.2 Innovation and Interruptions:

1. **Advanced Over-burden:** Unnecessary utilization of innovation, for example, cell phones and virtual entertainment, can upset equilibrium and concentration.
2. **Data Over-burden:** The steady inundation of data and warnings can overpower people.

2.3 Overcommitment:

1. **An excessive number of Commitments:** Overcommitting to different obligations and commitments can prompt burnout.
2. **Trouble Saying No:** Certain individuals battle to define limits and say no when fundamental.

2.4 Absence of Prioritization:

1. **Prioritization Difficulties:** Trouble in figuring out what is most significant in life can prompt irregularity.
2. **Absence of Objective Setting:** Without clear objectives, testing to pursue choices line up with one's qualities and needs.

2.5 Wellbeing Disregard:

1. **Unfortunate Taking care of oneself:** Disregarding physical and psychological wellness can bring about an absence of energy and prosperity.
2. **Unfortunate Things to do:** Undesirable propensities like an inactive way of life or a less than stellar eating routine can add to irregularity.

Procedures for Accomplishing Equilibrium
3.1 Self-Reflection:

1. **Characterize Your Qualities:** Distinguish your basic beliefs and the main thing to you throughout everyday life.
2. **Put forth Clear Objectives:** Put forth unambiguous and feasible objectives for different parts of your life.

3.2 Using time effectively:

1. **Focus on Assignments:** Use time usage procedures to focus on errands in view of significance and cutoff times.
2. **Delegate Whenever the situation allows:** Representative undertakings that others can deal with, saving your time for additional basic matters.

3.3 Work-Life Incorporation:

1. **Adaptable Work Plans:** Investigate adaptable work courses of action, like remote work or strategic scheduling, to more readily incorporate work and individual life.
2. **Limit Setting:** Lay out clear limits among work and individual chance to forestall business related pressure from influencing your own life.

3.4 Advanced Detox:

1. **Planned Innovation Breaks:** Assign explicit times during the day for browsing messages and utilizing computerized gadgets.
2. **Turn off Before Bed:** Make a sans tech sleep time routine to further develop rest quality.

3.5 Pressure The executives:

1. **Care and Reflection:** Practice care and contemplation to diminish pressure and upgrade profound equilibrium.

2. **Actual work:** Take part in normal active work, like yoga or running, to deliver pressure and lift by and large prosperity.

3.6 Taking care of oneself:

1. **Focus on Wellbeing:** Set aside a few minutes for customary activity, a reasonable eating routine, and satisfactory rest.
2. **Self-Sympathy:** Be thoughtful to yourself and practice self-empathy while confronting difficulties or misfortunes.

3.7 Figure out how to Say No:

1. **Put down Stopping points:** Figure out how to define limits and say no when important to forestall overcommitment.
2. **Particular Responsibility:** Spotlight on exercises and responsibilities that line up with your qualities and needs.

3.8 Look for Help:

1. **Contact Others:** Offer your objectives and difficulties with believed companions or relatives who can offer help and responsibility.
2. **Proficient Assistance:** Consider looking for direction from a specialist or holistic mentor to address explicit difficulties or hindrances.

Methodologies for Explicit Life Regions
4.1 Balance between serious and fun activities:

1. **Put down Stopping points:** Obviously characterize work hours and stick to them to make a solid work-life limit.
2. **Enjoy Normal Reprieves:** Integrate brief breaks into your business day to re-energize and keep up with center.

4.2 Family and Connections:

1. **Quality Time:** Distribute quality time for friends and family, liberated from interruptions or innovation.
2. **Correspondence:** Keep up with transparent correspondence with relatives to address any worries or clashes.

4.3 Wellbeing and Health:

1. **Customary Check-Ups:** Timetable normal clinical check-ups to screen your wellbeing and address any worries quickly.
2. **Comprehensive Health:** Embrace an all encompassing way to deal with wellbeing, including physical, mental, and close to home prosperity.

4.4 Self-improvement:

1. **Persistent Learning:** Put resources into self-improvement through perusing, courses, or studios to extend your insight and abilities.
2. **Self-Reflection:** Routinely ponder your self-improvement venture and change your objectives on a case by case basis.

4.5 Recreation and Leisure activities:

1. **Plan Recreation Time:** Devote time in your timetable for leisure activities and exercises you appreciate.
2. **Separate:** While taking part in relaxation exercises, detach from work and innovation to drench yourself completely.

Keeping up with Equilibrium Over the long haul
5.1 Intermittent Appraisal:

1. **Consistently Survey Objectives:** Occasionally evaluate your objectives and needs to guarantee they stay lined up with your qualities.
2. **Change depending on the situation:** change your procedures and needs as conditions change.

5.2 Self-Empathy:

1. **Embrace Flaw:** Comprehend that equilibrium doesn't mean flawlessness. There will be seasons of awkwardness, and that is not a problem.
2. **Taking care of oneself:** Focus on taking care of oneself to fabricate strength and return from difficulties.

5.3 Encouraging group of people:

1. **Rest on Others:** Go ahead and backing and direction from companions, family, or experts when required.
2. **Offer Help:** Be available to offering backing to others in your organization who might be battling with balance.

5.4 Care and Appreciation:

1. **Practice Care:** Consistently practice care to remain present and value life's minutes.
2. **Develop Appreciation:** Develop a feeling of appreciation for the equilibrium and satisfaction you experience.

8.1 Balancing work and personal life for overall equilibrium.

In the present speedy world, accomplishing a harmony among work and individual life has turned into a fundamental worry for some people. The requests of current vocations and the rising network empowered by innovation frequently obscure the lines among expert and individual life. This complete aide investigates the significance of accomplishing a harmony among work and individual life, the difficulties individuals face in keeping up with balance, and commonsense systems to lead a more agreeable and satisfying life.

Understanding the Meaning of Balance between fun and serious activities

1.1 Physical and Emotional well-being:

1. **Diminished Pressure:** A healthy lifestyle decreases feelings of anxiety, prompting better physical and emotional well-being.
2. **Worked on Prosperity:** Accomplishing harmony improves by and large prosperity and life fulfillment.

1.2 Improving Connections:

1. **Quality Time:** Adjusting work and individual life guarantees that you possess quality energy for friends and family, encouraging more grounded connections.
2. **Close to home Association:** A healthy lifestyle permits you to be genuinely present with loved ones.

1.3 Expert Achievement:

1. **Further developed Efficiency:** Equilibrium prompts expanded efficiency and imagination in the working environment.
2. **Diminished Burnout:** Forestalling business related burnout guarantees long haul profession achievement.

1.4 Individual Satisfaction:

1. **Chasing after Interests:** Equilibrium permits time for individual interests and interests, adding to a feeling of satisfaction.

2. **Life Improvement:** A balanced life prompts self-improvement and self-disclosure.

Normal Difficulties to Accomplishing Balance between fun and serious activities

2.1 Long Working Hours:

1. **Exhaust:** Requesting position frequently require long working hours, allowing for individual life.
2. **Strain to Play out:** The strain to meet work assumptions can prompt disregard of individual life.

2.2 Innovation and Availability:

1. **Computerized Over-burden:** Innovation empowers steady network, making it trying to disengage from work.
2. **Limit Obscuring:** The line among work and individual life becomes obscured because of the utilization of innovation.

2.3 Overcommitment:

1. **Such a large number of Commitments:** Overcommitment to different obligations and exercises can prompt lopsidedness.
2. **Trouble Saying No:** A few people battle to define limits and decline extra responsibilities.

2.4 Absence of Using time effectively:

1. **Dawdling:** Unfortunate time usage abilities can bring about stalling and an absence of equilibrium.
2. **Unfocused Work:** Wasteful work propensities can broaden work hours and spill into individual time.

2.5 Culpability and Assumptions:

1. **Culpability Over Prioritization:** Responsibility can emerge when people focus on private life over work.
2. **Outer Assumptions:** Society and work environment societies might put unreasonable demands on people to focus on work.

Procedures for Accomplishing Balance between serious and fun activities

3.1 Focus on and Put down Stopping points:

1. **Distinguish Needs:** Explain your guiding principle and recognize the main thing to you in both your expert and individual life.
2. **Put down Stopping points:** Lay out clear limits among work and individual life to keep work from infringing on your own time.

3.2 Compelling Using time productively:

1. **Focus on Undertakings:** Use time usage procedures, like the Eisenhower Grid, to focus on errands in light of significance and desperation.
2. **Time Obstructing:** Designate explicit time blocks for business related assignments and individual exercises to keep up with balance.

3.3 Figure out how to Say No:

1. **Survey Responsibilities:** Assess your ongoing responsibilities and be specific about taking on new ones.
2. **Pleasant Decay:** Figure out how to decline extra responsibilities cordially and emphatically when fundamental.

3.4 Think about the big picture before attacking the details:

1. **Put down certain boundaries:** Lay out limits on working hours and use strategies like the Pomodoro Strategy to work in engaged, concentrated explodes.
2. **Delegate Undertakings:** Representative assignments when conceivable to diminish your responsibility and save time for individual life.

3.5 Innovation and Availability The executives:

1. **Computerized Detox:** Timetable normal breaks from innovation to disengage from business related messages and notices.
2. **Work Email Arrangements:** Lay out strategies for work messages beyond available time to set clear assumptions.

3.6 Taking care of oneself:

1. **Focus on Wellbeing:** Focus on taking care of oneself by consolidating customary activity, a reasonable eating regimen, and satisfactory rest into your daily schedule.
2. **Mental Health:** Participate in care and unwinding methods to oversee pressure and work on mental prosperity.

3.7 Seek after Interests and Leisure activities:

1. **Plan Recreation Time:** Devote time in your timetable for side interests and exercises you appreciate.
2. **Disengage:** While taking part in recreation exercises, detach from work and innovation to submerge yourself completely.

3.8 Look for Help:

1. **Share with Friends and family:** Offer your objectives and difficulties with believed companions or relatives who can offer help and responsibility.
2. **Proficient Assistance:** Consider looking for direction from a specialist or holistic mentor to address explicit difficulties or obstructions.

Keeping up with Balance between serious and fun activities Over the long haul

4.1 Occasional Assessment:

1. **Consistently Survey Objectives:** Intermittently evaluate your objectives and needs to guarantee they stay lined up with your qualities.
2. **Change on a case by case basis:** change your procedures and needs as conditions change.

4.2 Self-Empathy:

1. **Embrace Blemish:** Comprehend that balance between serious and fun activities doesn't mean flawlessness. There will be seasons of unevenness, and that is completely fine.
2. **Taking care of oneself:** Focus on taking care of oneself to construct strength and return from mishaps.

4.3 Encouraging group of people:

1. **Rest on Others:** Go ahead and backing and direction from companions, family, or experts when required.
2. **Offer Help:** Be available to offering backing to others in your organization who might be battling with balance between fun and serious activities.

4.4 Care and Appreciation:

1. **Practice Care:** Routinely practice care to remain present and value life's minutes.
2. **Develop Appreciation:** Develop a feeling of appreciation for the equilibrium and satisfaction you experience.

8.2 Stress management techniques for improved balance.

In our high speed and requesting world, stress has turned into a practically steady friend for some individuals. The adverse consequences of stress can negatively affect both our physical and mental prosperity, upsetting the equilibrium we look for in our lives. This thorough aide plans to investigate the meaning of pressure the board in accomplishing in general equilibrium and prosperity. We will dig into different pressure the board procedures and systems that can assist people with recovering control, decrease feelings of anxiety, and reestablish harmony in their lives.

Figuring out the Effect of Weight on Equilibrium

1.1 Actual Wellbeing:

1. **Hormonal Reaction:** Ongoing pressure sets off the arrival of stress chemicals like cortisol, which can prompt weight gain, cardiovascular issues, and resistant framework concealment.
2. **Muscle Strain:** Stress frequently appears as muscle pressure and solidness, adding to actual distress.

1.2 Mental Prosperity:

1. **Mental Weakness:** Delayed pressure can disable mental capability, influencing navigation, memory, and focus.
2. **Close to home Effect:** Stress can prompt mind-set problems like tension and sadness, further upsetting profound equilibrium.

1.3 Relational Connections:

1. **Correspondence Difficulties:** High-feelings of anxiety can prompt correspondence breakdowns, clashes, and stressed connections.
2. **Absence of Presence:** Stress can keep people from being completely present in their associations with friends and family, influencing the nature of connections.

1.4 Balance between fun and serious activities:

1. **Overpower:** Stress can prompt business related burnout, making it trying to keep a sound balance between fun and serious activities.
2. **Loss of Happiness:** High-feelings of anxiety can reduce one's capacity to track down pleasure and fulfillment in both work and individual life.

Techniques for Viable Pressure The executives
2.1 Care and Reflection:

1. **Care Practices:** Participate in care works out, like profound breathing, reflection, and moderate muscle unwinding, to remain present and diminish pressure.
2. **Careful Living:** Apply care standards to day to day existence by zeroing in on each undertaking in turn and relishing the current second.

2.2 Actual work:

1. **Normal Activity:** Integrate standard actual work into your everyday practice, like yoga, running, swimming, or moving, to deliver pressure lessening endorphins.

2. **Mind-Body Practices:** Investigate mind-body rehearses like Kendo or Qigong, which consolidate development and contemplation to mitigate pressure.

2.3 Using time effectively:

1. **Prioritization:** Use time usage strategies to focus on errands, put forth sensible objectives, and stay away from overcommitment.
2. **Time Obstructing:** Apportion explicit time blocks for business related undertakings and individual exercises to keep up with balance.

2.4 Unwinding Methods:

1. **Profound Relaxing:** Practice profound breathing activities, for example, diaphragmatic breathing or box breathing, to enact the body's unwinding reaction.
2. **Representation:** Utilize directed symbolism and perception strategies to make mental pictures of quiet and unwinding.

2.5 Mental Procedures:

1. **Positive Insistences:** Utilize positive confirmations to counter bad self-talk and develop a more hopeful mentality.
2. **Mental Social Treatment (CBT):** Consider CBT, an organized psychotherapy

approach, to recognize and challenge silly contemplations that add to pressure.

2.6 Social Help:

1. **Looking for Help:** Feel free to out to companions, family, or psychological well-being experts for help and direction.

2. **Bunch Exercises:** Take part in bunch exercises or care groups to associate with other people who might have comparative stressors.

2.7 Taking care of oneself:

1. **Focus on Wellbeing:** Focus on taking care of oneself by consolidating standard activity, a decent eating regimen, and sufficient rest into your daily practice.
2. **Stress Decrease Customs:** Make pressure decrease ceremonies, like cleaning up, perusing, or taking part in imaginative leisure activities.

2.8 Time for Recreation and Side interests:

1. **Plan Recreation Time:** Devote time in your timetable for side interests and exercises you appreciate.
2. **Disengage:** While taking part in recreation exercises, separate from work and innovation to drench yourself completely.

2.9 Confident Correspondence:

1. **Put down Stopping points:** Practice confident correspondence to define clear limits with associates, companions, and family in regards to your time and cutoff points.
2. **Express Requirements:** Obviously express your necessities and worries in relational connections to keep pressure from developing.

2.10 Expert Assistance:

1. **Remedial Help:** In the event that pressure is overpowering, consider looking for proficient assistance from a specialist or guide who can give customized methodologies and backing.
2. **Drug:** at times, medicine endorsed by a medical services proficient might be important to oversee pressure related side effects.

Integrating Pressure The board into Day to day existence
3.1 Wake-up routines:

1. **Careful Beginning:** Start your day with a couple of seconds of care, zeroing in on your breath and setting a positive expectation for the afternoon.
2. **Actual work:** Integrate a concise morning work-out daily practice, like extending or yoga, to support your energy and lessen pressure.

3.2 Pressure Busting Breaks:

1. **Small scale Contemplations:** Enjoy short reprieves over the course of the day to rehearse little reflections or profound breathing activities to ease pressure.
2. **Nature Association:** Put shortly in nature, regardless of whether it's simply a concise stroll outside, to re-energize and diminish pressure.

3.3 Time Obstructing:

1. **Organized Work Time:** Carry out time hindering for business related errands, guaranteeing committed center during those periods.
2. **Devoted Individual Time:** Comparably, designate explicit time blocks for individual exercises and unwinding.

3.4 Careful Eating:

1. **Smart dieting Propensities:** Practice careful eating by relishing your feasts, staying away from interruptions, and going with nutritious decisions to help your prosperity.
2. **Hydration:** Remain hydrated over the course of the day, as drying out can add to pressure and weariness.

3.5 Night Wind-Down:

1. **Advanced Detox:** Cutoff screen time and openness to computerized gadgets at night to further develop rest quality and lessen pressure.
2. **Unwinding Customs:** Lay out unwinding ceremonies before sleep time, like delicate extending, perusing, or rehearsing appreciation.

Long haul Pressure The board and Anticipation
4.1 Occasional Evaluation:

1. **Customary Self-Reflection:** Occasionally evaluate your feelings of anxiety, triggers, and the viability of your pressure the board methods.
2. **Change and Adjust:** change your pressure the board techniques as your life conditions change.

4.2 Care and Appreciation:

1. **Everyday Practice:** Proceed with day to day care and appreciation practices to keep
   up with profound equilibrium and strength.
2. **Journaling:** Keep a pressure diary to follow your stressors, responses, and progress in overseeing pressure.

4.3 Keep up with Social Associations:

1. **Sustain Connections:** Keep on putting time and exertion in supporting and keeping up with positive connections.
2. **Correspondence:** Practice transparent correspondence with friends and family to forestall clashes and errors.

4.4 Consistent Learning and Development:

1. **Long lasting Learning:** Embrace deep rooted advancing by chasing after interests,
   obtaining new abilities, and testing yourself mentally.
2. **Versatility:** Develop flexibility and strength to adapt to life's progressions and vulnerabilities successfully.